PSYCHOANALYTIC INQ

A Topical Journal for Mental Health Professionals

Volume 19	1999	Number 4

Attachment Research and Psychoanalysis:
1. Theoretical Considerations

STATEMENT OF OWNERSHIP, MANAGEMENT, AND CIRCULATION

Date of filing: October 1, 1999

Title of publication: *Psychoanalytic Inquiry*   Publication No.: 0735-1690

Issue Frequency: Five times a year   No. Issues Published Annually: 5

Annual subscription price: $73 (1999)

Location of known office of publication: 810 E. 10th Street, Lawrence, KS 66044-8897

Contact person: Theresa Pickel   Phone: 785-843-1235

Location of headquarters or general business office of publisher: 810 E. 10th Street,
   Lawrence, KS 66044-8897

Editor: Joseph D. Lichtenberg, M.D., l6l6 18th St. NW, Washington DC 20009

Managing Editor: Nancy Liguori, 101 West Street, Hillsdale, NJ 07642

No known bondholders, mortgagees, or other security holders

Issue date for circulation data below: June/July 1999

	Average no. copies each issue during preceding 12 months	Actual no. copies single issue published nearest to filing date
Total no. copies	1772	1880
Paid and/or requested circulation:	945	942
Other classes mailed through the UPPS	204	182
Total paid and/or requested circulation	1149	1124
Free distribution by mail	50	0
Other classes mailed through the UPPS	22	21
Free distribution outside mail	14	13
Total free distribution	87	34
Total distribution	1236	1158
Copies not distributed	536	722
Total:	1772	1880
Percent paid/and/or requested circulation	93.0	97.1

For the publisher: _____

Paul E. Stepansky, Ph.D., Managing Director

Dedication

THESE TWO VOLUMES on attachment theory and research are dedicated to the memory of Mary D. Saltar Ainsworth, who died on March 21, 1999.

Mary Saltar Ainsworth, as I think of her over our 40 years of acquaintance, was large—large physically, large in heart, and very, very large in accomplishment. The theory of attachment we document in these two volumes of *Psychoanalytic Inquiry* could not have come about without her brilliance and simplicity, a rare combination. If Mary wanted to see if Bowlby's ideas were correct, she went where she could observe the evidence. Observing, for Mary, meant looking with the most sensitive powers of perception at the whole of child rearing in Uganda. Simplicity meant that if she wanted to observe responses to separation in an urban culture, she would set up a test situation that could be standardized and confirmed by others. Look, study, document—not coldly, not experience distant, but right where we live as humans. Thus Mary chose for her book *Infancy in Uganda* the subtitle *Infant Care and the Growth of Love*. Mary's writing reveals her freedom from the distraction of all the psychoanalytic arguments about drive theory that swirled around Bowlby. She simply went to the heart of the matter—the caregiver and the child and their interplay. We psychoanalysts now reap the harvest of her freedom to explore. In an inscription to the Uganda book Mary gave me on its publication, she wrote: "I hope you enjoy this. I enjoyed writing it." Mary knew how to enjoy—to play. We lose her in death but, as she taught us, attachment is about the mastery of danger and loss.

Joseph D. Lichtenberg, M.D.
Editor-in-Chief

Prologue

W E ARE AT A PRIVILEGED MOMENT in the study of the relationship between attachment theory and psychoanalysis. Psychoanalysis has always had close links to developmental psychology, being enriched by developmental theory and research and, in turn, contributing to and participating in developmental investigations. This close relationship between attachment and developmental psychology has been enriched and extended over the past two decades by the identification of several different patterns of attachment between infant and the caregiver (Ainsworth et al., 1978) and of the representational processes that are the "likely mediators of differences in parental caregiving" (Hesse, 1999, p. 395; Main, Kaplan, and Cassidy, 1985). Attachment theory and research initially emerged from the clinical observations of the psychoanalyst John Bowlby, who identified the proclivity to form affectional bonds with significant others who are likely to promote the individual's safety and survival as pivotal to human motivation. He theorized that this affectional bond serves the evolutionary function of maintaining the infant's proximity to the mother in the face of separation, and that the child will inevitably develop strategies to regulate proximity to the caretaker, strategies shaped in part by the nature of the caretaker's response to the child's distress at separation and attempts to reestablish proximity (Bowlby, 1969, 1973, 1988). Bowlby's delineation of the attachment motivational system was enhanced and extended through considerable experimental investigation, first by Mary Ainsworth (Ainsworth et al., 1978, 1985) and later by a host of other investigators, some of whom have contributed to this two-issue series on psychoanalysis and attachment theory and research. Most readers of this prologue are already familiar with the basic tenets of attachment theory and research, but for a comprehensive overview, see the papers by Fonagy and Hesse and Main (this issue).

This creative rapproachment or synthesis between psychoanalysis and developmental psychology, particularly expressed in attachment research, has led, for example, during the past several years to major panels on attachment theory and its clinical implications at the meetings of both the American Psychoanalytic Association and the Division of Psychoanalysis (Division 39) of the American Psychological Association. In addition, a number of recent articles have assessed the divergence and convergence between attachment research and psychoanalytic theory (Silverman, 1991, 1998; Slade and Aber, 1992; Diamond and Blatt, 1994). The synthesis of concepts from psychoanalysis and attachment theory have led to a more comprehensive understanding of the representational world (Diamond and Blatt, 1994), affect regulation (Silverman, 1998), and aspects of the therapeutic process (Dozier, 1990, 1993; Fonagy, 1991; Holmes, 1993a, 1996, 1999; Farber, Lippert, and Nevas, 1995; Slade, 1999). The application of constructs from attachment theory to clinical phenomena has contributed substantially to an understanding of the developmental origins of various forms of psychopathology, including anxiety (Cassidy, 1995), depression (Blatt and Homann, 1992), personality disorders (Fonagy, 1991; Patrick et al., 1994; Fonagy et al., 1995; Fonagy et al., 1996; Allen, Hauser, and Borman-Spurrell, 1996), and dissociative disorders (Liotti, 1995; Main and Morgan, 1996; Hesse and Main, this issue). Attachment between infant and caregiver, the biologically stable proclivity of the infant to form affectional bonds with caregivers (Bowlby, 1969, 1973, 1988), has also contributed extensively to the emerging new field of developmental psychopathology (see for example Cicchetti, 1995, 1997), and these observations are now beginning to have a major impact on the theory and practice of psychoanalysis and psychoanalytic psychotherapy (e.g., Fonagy, 1991; Fonagy et al., 1995; Holmes, 1993a,b, 1995, 1996; Slade, 1999).

John Bowlby clearly envisioned such a creative dialogue between clinicians and research investigators. He believed that attachment theory, born in psychoanalytic observations in the consulting room and developed further through investigations with nonclinical samples, would be revised and expanded by research in both normal and clinical settings. In a relatively late work, *A Secure Base* (1988), Bowlby reflected on the clinical implications of attachment theory and research and expressed his disappointment that attachment theory, which had its genesis in object relations orientation and in the psychoanalytic treatment of severely disturbed patients, had never been embraced by psychoanalytic clinicians.

> It is a little unexpected that, whereas attachment theory was formulated by a clinician for use in the diagnosis and treatment of seriously disturbed patients and families, its usage hitherto has been mainly to promote research in developmental psychology. . . . Whilst I welcome the findings of this research as enormously extending our understanding of personality development and psychopathology, and thus as of the greatest clinical relevance, it nonetheless has been disappointing that clinicians have been so slow to test the theory's use [p. ix].

We have designed these two issues on the relationship between psychoanalysis and attachment theory and research with the hope of contributing to the creative dialogue between psychoanalytic clinicians and attachment investigators that Bowlby envisioned. The first issue addresses the theoretical implications of attachment research for psychoanalytic theory, with a focus on the convergences and divergences between the two theoretical positions. The second issue explores the clinical implications of attachment research and how it can contribute to a psychoanalytic understanding of various forms of psychopathology and the treatment process.

These two issues of *Psychoanalytic Inquiry* represent yet another chapter in articulating relationships between the two theoretical traditions (psychoanalysis and developmental theory) but also between clinical practice and empirical investigation. This effort at interdisciplinary integration can sometimes provoke bitter polemic, such as that which led to Bowlby being ostracized by the British Psychoanalytic Institute after Bowlby, in an early paper, "The Nature of the Child's Tie to Its Mother" (Bowlby, 1958), posited that the attachment behavioral system is a central motivational force and that mother–infant attachment is an irreducible medium of human interaction. These formulations were initially viewed as anathema to psychoanalytic thought predominant at the time which maintained allegiance to a dual drive reduction theory of psychological development, despite the fact that a number of prominent psychoanalysts, especially in the British Psychoanalytic Society, were formulating theories giving increased primacy to the need for and the orientation toward objects. It is unclear to what extent Bowlby's formulation of the attachment system—the desire to form affectional bonds with significant others as a biologically stable motivational force—was continuous or discontinuous with the object relations tradition emerging at that time, particularly the concepts of primary object seeking (Fairbairn, 1952), primary love (Balint, 1952), and the importance of primary object relations both real and fantasied (Klein, 1946). For those who believe that Bowlby's formulations represented an inevitable development of aspects of psychoanalysis and particularly psychoanalytic object relations theory, Bowlby's ostracism from the psychoanalytic community is considered one of the most "dreadful, shameful and regrettable chapters in the history of psychoanalysis" (Grotstein, quoted in Holmes, 1995, p. 26). The ostracism of Bowlby may have also been the consequence of Bowlby's reliance on theory and research from evolutionary biology and developmental psychology as some of the theoretical support for his formulations. Some argue that Bowlby's subsequent repudiation of his psychoanalytic roots may have been more reactive than substantive in that it served to highlight the uniqueness and divergence of Bowlby's formulations with classic psychoanalytic thought rather than how it maintained continuity with prior object relations formulations (Fonagy, this issue). Bowlby, however, gave the impression of considerable concern about his alienation from the psychoanalytic establishment and indicated that he viewed attachment theory as a natural extension of psychoanalytic thought. One of us (SJB) had the very good fortune in February 1989 to have John Bowlby as the discussant for a presentation he made at the Tavistock Center. Subsequent to that presentation, as Blatt was invited into Bowlby's office at the Tavistock, for what turned out to be a delightful meeting that lasted for over 2 hours, Bowlby's first question as they entered his office was. "Do you think of me as a psychoanalyst?"

Despite the controversial beginning of attachment theory within psychoanalysis, developments in both psychoanalysis and attachment theory have increasingly brought these two traditions into synchrony. As psychoanalysts increasingly consider the potential contributions of neurobiology, ethology, linguistics, narrative theory, and cognitive or information theory to psychoanalysis, they have to increasingly reconsider the value of attachment theory, which in its own right has attempted to encompass many of these other areas of inquiry. Indeed, major shifts in psychoanalytic thought over the last 30 years have paralleled those in attachment theory and research, including: (1) the reevaluation of the relative importance of the early mother–infant relationship (of preoedipal, as well as oedipal, factors) and the salience of early experience with attachment figures in the formation of personality and psychic structure (e.g., Kernberg, 1975; Mahler, Pine, and Bergman, 1975; Loewald, 1980; Lichtenberg, 1985; Stern, 1985); (2) a reexamination and expansion of the concept of motivation, with some theorists going beyond the dual-drive theory to a consideration of attachment as a primary motivator (Lichtenberg, 1992; Westen, 1997), while others, who retain allegiance to the dual drive theory, develop a more finely nuanced and complex understanding of the relationships between drive, affect, and object (e.g., Loewald, 1980; Kernberg, 1990); (3) a reconceptualization of the psychoanalytic process as narrative construction in which historical and narrative truth, current experience, and retrospective reconstruction are inextricably intertwined (e.g., Schafer, 1992; Hanly, 1996); (4) the increasing attention to the operationalization of psychoanalytic concepts and to empirical research on psychoanalytic process and outcome (e.g., Wallerstein, 1986; Blatt and Ford, 1994; Blatt et al., 1996), with particular attention to instruments that measure psychoanalytic change such as the Adult Attachment Interview (AAI; Main and Goldwyn, 1994), which assesses the structure and content of narratives about early life experiences (Fonagy et al., 1996), and The Object Representation Inventory (ORI; e.g., Blatt et al., 1996), which assesses the structure and content of mental representations of self and significant others.

Just as the psychoanalytic community is reconsidering the value of attachment theory and research for enriching and revising aspects of psychoanalytic theory and process, so are attachment investigators reconsidering the relationship of attachment theory to psychoanalysis. The development of the AAI, which links the quality and form of narrative discourse in adults to parent–child attachment patterns in infancy, has raised issues about processes of internalization and the nature of the internal world that are central to psychoanalytic inquiry. The analysis of narrative discourse on the AAI provides a window into the representational world and particularly to the nature of internal working models of early attachment relationships. Internal working models are viewed as rules and expectations that govern attachment behavior, as well as the nature of representations of self and attachment figures, and in this regard converge with psychoanalytic concepts of self and object representations (Main et al., 1985; Diamond and Blatt, 1994). Both internal working models in attachment theory (Bowlby, 1969, 1988) and self-object-affect units in psychoanalytic theory (Kernberg, 1975) represent the internalization of early affectively-charged experiences with significant others, and their translation into internal representational models or structures. Bowlby (1988) redefined an "internal object as a working, or representational model of an attachment figure" (p. 151), and stated that "within an attachment framework, the concept of working model of an attachment figure is [sic] in many respects equivalent to and replaces, the traditional psychoanalytic concept of internal object" (p. 120). Bowlby's articulation of the overlap between the concept of working models of attachment and psychoanalytic notions of self and object representations has been echoed in psychoanalytic thought as psychoanalysts increasingly concern themselves with an exploration of cognitive-affective aspects of representational processes and their role as mediators of interpersonal relationships.

Internal working models not only systematically represent attachment figures and self, but they also organize strategies for regulating affect. The strategies of affect regulation that grow out of different attachment patterns have been conceptualized as defensive strategies designed to maximize proximity to and contact with the caretaker (Cassidy, 1994). Thus, the investigation of internal working models of attachment has led attachment researchers to formulate a theory of defensive functioning that also echoes psychoanalytic formulations that defenses are created as part of the developmental process as affects inevitably become associated with the representation of desired and feared states in relation to others. The attachment view of defenses differs from the classical psychoanalytic view in that attachment focuses on outer threat (i.e., rejecting, inconsistent, or traumatizing parenting) rather than the press of unmanageable affects or impulses as the precipitant for defensive functioning or the formation of defenses; however, both theories emphasize the centrality of defenses for personality organization and symptom constructions. But intense affects are provoked by difficult and disruptive parenting, and therefore, the defensive responses are often in reaction to intense affects of desire and anger. Further, in both attachment and psychoanalytic theory, defenses serve to protect the individual from overwhelming forces and internal conflicts, by limiting the access of these forces and conflicts to consciousness. In psychoanalysis, defenses are linked to these threatening and potentially overwhelming forces and internal conflicts, while in attachment theory defenses are linked to the vicissitudes of interactions with the attachment object and to the activation or deactivation of the attachment system that serve the adaptive function of survival by insuring proximity to the caretaker.

The purpose of these two issues is to deepen and advance the already substantial dialogue between attachment theory and psychoanalysis. Some of the papers in this first issue, particularly the one by Fonagy, emphasize points of contact and convergence between psychoanalytic and attachment theory; while other papers acknowledge points of overlap, they also emphasize what is distinct and unique about each theory, such as the contributions by Levy and Blatt on the representational world or by Hesse and Main on the disorganized/disoriented attachment pattern. Other papers, such as those by Lyons-Ruth and by George and Solomon, offer perspectives on caretaking and on early parent–child transactions that use both attachment and psychoanalytic theories as springboards for further theoretical innovation. Some of the papers, in their advance of attachment theory, pose a challenge to psychoanalytic concepts. All of the papers in this first issue, however, whether they emphasize points of contact or divergence, demonstrate that psychoanalysis and attachment theory can be complimentary and that the tension between the two traditions can provide the matrix for creative interchange and enrichment of both theories.

In the first paper in this issue, "Points of Contact and Divergence Between Psychoanaltyic and Attachment Theories: Is Psychoanalytic Theory Truly Different? Peter Fonagy offers a timely reconsideration of the areas of convergence between the two theories as well as a masterful integration of conceptions of psychoanalytic and attachment theory. Reframing the nature of the debate between psychoanalysts and attachment theorists, Fonagy states that, with a few exceptions (e.g., Lichtenberg, Eagle, Holmes), theorists in both camps have caricatured each other's theories by focusing on the weakest or most problematic aspects in ways that have blocked attempts at clarification and synthesis. Fonagy then provides a thoughtful clarification of distortions about attachment theory that have been perpetuated within psychoanalysis, grounding some of them in the psychoanalytic politics of the time and in the polarization that can occur during theory building. He reexamines some of the major objections that theorists from each tradition have levied against the other and how these objections are, in fact, examples of failure to consider the complex multifaceted nature of both traditions. These objections also tend to downplay areas of convergence such as their complementary views of the internal or representational world. In addition, Fonagy invites us to consider how Bowlby's formulation of a primary need for safety and physical caretaking, as key motivations for object seeking, provided a firm biological and evolutionary basis to the primary proclivity of infants to seek and relate to objects in reality and fantasy, long a hallmark of object relations theorists. What distinguishes Bowlby from the object relations theorists of his time, in Fonagy's view, is his exclusive focus on the sociobiological, rather than psychological, root of the infant's proclivity to seek proximity to and connectedness with the caretaker. While Bowlby may have exaggerated the importance of evolutionary considerations such as the physical need for safety and protection to emphasize what distinguished his theory from psychoanalytic object relations theory, he also provided psychoanalysis with a potentially unifying theory.

Additionally, Fonagy provides a comprehensive overview of the ways in which attachment theory and the attachment concept grew out of and is consistent with psychoanalytic traditions. By differentiating the construct of attachment from attachment theory and research, Fonagy invites us to reconsider how this construct has evolved in psychoanalytic thought both previous to and concurrent with the development of the concept of attachment as defined by Bowlby. Fonagy points out echoes of the concept of secure attachment in Erikson's basic trust, Bion's containment, and Klein's depressive position. It is here that Fonagy makes creative theoretical integrations that enhance our understanding of both theories. He sees, for example, Bion's containment, the process by which the caretaker comprehends and metabolizes the infant's affective states into tolerable and thinkable experiences, as the psychological analogue of the infant's proclivity to seek proximity to the caretaker. In addition, Fonagy reexamines attachment theory and the various categories of attachment in the light of Klein's concepts of the paranoid-schizoid and depressive position. Insecure attachment, which involves a lack of coherent representations and inconsistent experiences with the caretaker, is compared with the paranoid-schizoid position in which the relationship with the caretaker is split into persecutory and idealized aspects. Secure attachment, by contrast, which involves the capacity to represent the caretaker in an integrated and coherent manner and the capacity to integrate and reflect on positive and negative aspects of these representations, has much in common with the depressive position, which presupposes the capacity to develop an integrated image of the loved and hated aspects of the parents, and a corresponding integration of the self.

Fonagy thus finds original and imaginative points of intersection between attachment theory and psychoanalysis that amplify and enrich our understanding of both traditions. An example of such creative synthesis and integration is Fonagy's concept of reflective function, or the capacity to perceive, comprehend, and reason about the mental states of self and others, which draws on and integrates attachment, cognitive-developmental and psychoanalytic theories. Reflective function evolved in part from Main's (1991) conceptualization of metacognitive monitoring, or the capacity to actively monitor and reflect on one's own processes of thinking and recall, as a cornerstone of secure attachment. Fonagy's theory of reflective function enhances and extends our understanding of attachment security. According to Fonagy, secure attachment provides the basis for the development of the psychological capacity for awareness and exploration of the mental states of self and others, while insecure attachment presupposes a defensive exclusion of the mental contents of the other (avoidant attachment), over involvement with the mind of the other (ambivalent attachment), or hyperattunement to the mental states of the other to the neglect of one's own mental states (disorganized/disoriented attachment).

Reflective function is also consistent with psychoanalytic concepts including Klein's (1935) depressive position which implies the individual's capacity to reflect on and integrate loving and hateful feelings toward the object, Bion's (1967) containment as the process by which mother transforms raw, unmanageable affect into tolerable, thinkable experiences; Winnicott's (1960) notion of the true (versus the false) self as brought into being by the mother's recognition of and vibrant responsivity to the full range of the child's internal states, and Hartmann's (1958) concept of self-reflectivity and intentionality.

In their paper, "Second-Generation Effects of Unresolved Trauma in Nonmaltreating Parents: Dissociated, Frightened, and Threatening Parental Behavior," Erik Hesse and Mary Main stress what is distinctive and unique in attachment theory both in its theoretical foundations and in its recent research developments. They focus on the proliferation of research on the disorganized/disoriented attachment category in infants, which in multiple studies has been linked to the AAI classification indicating that an individual (in this case the parent) is unresolved with respect to trauma and loss, and most recently to specific parental-child transactions observed naturalistically. The authors situate the discovery of the *disorganized* attachment category in the context of a succinct, but comprehensive overview of attachment theory and research in general, which includes a review of the nature and derivation of the three other *organized* attachment categories (e.g. secure, insecure-ambivalent and insecure-avoidant).

Hesse and Main begin by reaffirming the basic tenet of attachment theory: that Bowlby's unique contribution was to recognize the ethological significance of the proclivity to form enduring attachments to protective caretaking figures—a proclivity activated originally in our evolutionary history by the necessity of escaping from predators, and gradually transformed via natural selection during the course of human development into the biologically stable attachment behavioral system. According to Hesse and Main, attachment theory represents a convergence of object relations theory with evolutionary biology in that it stresses the primacy of object seeking and the intrinsic importance of early parent–infant interactions, but locates the motivation for the infant's object-seeking proclivity primarily in the necessity for survival, which in nomadic ground-dwelling primates involves the search for the attachment figure, rather than for a specific place or den. Attachment is inevitably intertwined with the activation of fear which causes the infant to seek the attachment figure as a haven of safety—thus, fear is an affect that is at the heart of the attachment behavioral system and its activation. It is not surprising, therefore, that much recent attachment research has investigated the disorganized/ disoriented attachment behaviors that result when the attachment figure, who should be the infant's solution to fear, becomes simultaneously a source of alarm.

Indeed, Hesse and Main see the evolution of disorganized/ disoriented attachment behaviors as the logical outcome of the simultaneous inhibition and activation of the attachment behavioral system itself. In situations where the attachment figure, ordinarily the haven of safety, is the source of threat, the infant exhibits behaviors which are both disorganized (e.g., contradictory and chaotic) and disoriented (e.g., not oriented to person or place). The simultaneous activation of the attachment behavioral system, that leads the infant to approach the parent—together with the escape (fear) system, that activates flight, results in contradictory and chaotic infant behaviors such as approaching the parent and then freezing or stilling, or simultaneously smiling at and attacking the attachment figure—behaviors that represent the internal chaos that results when the attachment figure itself becomes the source of fear.

A number of studies have shown a highly disproportional percentage of disorganized infants in maltreating samples, as would be expected on the basis of the above hypothesis. In this paper Hesse and Main additionally discuss the ways in which infant disorganized/ disoriented attachment is linked to unresolved trauma in the parent as assessed on the AAI both in high-risk groups, where there has been direct maltreatment of the child by the parent and in low-risk or non-maltreating families. It is the latter group that Hesse and Main investigate in this remarkable paper. Integrating theory and research, they illustrate how disorganized/disoriented attachment in infancy may result from parental lack of resolution of trauma and loss, as evidenced in linguistic slippages in narrative discourse on the AAI, such as talking about the deceased individual as though he or she were still alive, or exhibiting sudden and dramatic disfluencies, loss of memory or breaks in the narrative when discussing past abuse. Such unresolved status in the parents may be transmitted to the infant, not only through direct behavioral reenactment, but through the indirect, subtle behavioral and affective cues that devolve from the parent's often partially dissociated sense of an internal catastrophe around past traumatic experiences and losses. Thus, Hesse and Main show how a disorganized internal working model of attachment in the child may be shaped partly by internal processes in the parents that are experienced as traumatic even in low-risk (nonmaltreating) samples.

The paper breaks new theoretical and empirical ground by closing the transmission gap between unresolved past traumas and their internal representation in the parent and disorganized/ disoriented attachment behaviors in the infant in the absence of direct maltreatment or abuse. The authors present data derived from a coding system, entitled the Frightening, Frightened, Dissociated, Deferential, Sexualized and Disorganized Parental Behavior: A Coding System for Frightening Parent–infant interactions (Main and Hess, 1998), designed to assess frightening behaviors observed naturalistically in parent–child transactions such a play or feeding. This coding system, designated the FR coding system, encompasses several classes of parental behaviors including 1) predatory or threatening non-gamelike behaviors such as baring teeth, growling, clawing at or stalking the infant; 2) frightened or inhibited behaviors such as fearfully backing away from the infant as though he or she were a predator; 3) dissociated behaviors such as falling into trance-like states, moving in an asymmetrical or robotic manner; or 4) eroticized behaviors such as overly zealous caressing or kissing accompanied by seductive words, expressions or gestures. Intriguingly, Hesse and Main state that such behaviors are difficult to identify and classify because they are often fleeting and momentary, and hence thought to be derived from partially-dissociated memories or states in the parents. Indeed, the FR coding system provides empirical support for the idea that the internal representations of trauma in the parents are conveyed through subtle behaviors that devolve from parental fear and dissociation, and that in turn trigger the child's fright and dissociation. Parent-child transactions that fall under the rubric of frightened/frightening behaviors might be defined as traumatic in a cumulative sense.

Although Hesse and Main remain rooted in an attachment model that links internal working models to actual parental behaviors, they illustrate how mediating factors can enable a parent's past catastrophic history to be transmitted to the child not only through actual overt abuse, but through an accretion of interactions that constitute cumulative trauma, which is transmitted to the child and then expressed in infant disorganized behaviors and later in the child's catastrophic fantasies. Hesse and Main point out that behavioral disorganization which results from the simultaneous activation of proximity-seeking behavior and flight leads to a "positive feedback loop of escalating conflict and fear" that may be inherently pathogenic. The authors cite multiple studies which indicate that although by age 6, the behavioral disorganization is replaced by more organized, albeit controlling or punitive behaviors towards parents, the disorganization persists at the representational level. Children categorized as disorganized/ disoriented in infancy are observed in a number of studies to articulate catastrophic fantasies involving themes of violence, death, or severe illness or injury in their doll-play sequences or in their verbal responses to separation pictures or narratives in later childhood. Hesse and Main conclude that the disorganized/disoriented category may prefigure the development of psychopathology later in life, particularly when accompanied by temperamental predisposition or exposure to further trauma. The authors caution, however, that the specific pathways from disorganized/disoriented attachment in infancy to anxiety, dissociative, and/or borderline disorders in adulthood (with which the disorganized/ disoriented and unresolved for trauma and loss attachment categories have been associated in previous research) have yet to be delineated. Their elaboration of the disorganized/disoriented category in which there is a collapse of any coherent attachment strategy in infants, the predominance of catastrophic fantasies in childhood, and incoherent, fragmented or bizarre narratives in adulthood, potentially provides an empirically-grounded developmental perspective on these disorders and their transgenerational transmission.

In "Attachment Theory and Psychoanalysis: Further Differentiation Within Insecure Attachment Patterns," Kenneth Levy and Sidney Blatt cross-reference psychoanalytic concepts of self and object representations with the concept of internal working models of attachment in ways that advance our understanding of the representational world. The authors synthesize a large body of research with both clinical and nonclinical samples to delineate a developmental continuum from lower to higher representations both within and between the attachment categories. They begin with an overview and synthesis of psychoanalytic and attachment views of the representational world, delineating the attachment categories that have been identified in laboratory-based research on parent–child transactions and through analyses of narrative discourse on the AAI. They then review the social–psychological literature on romantic attachment relationships in adolescents and adults, conducted with self-report attachment questionnaires, and show how this literature, which tends to be neglected by both attachment and psychoanalytic theorists, potentially enhances our understanding of attachment categories and the representational processes that underlie them. Specifically, they delineate how a large range of studies with self-report instruments (such as the Bartholomew Attachment Questionnaire [the BAQ] have enabled investigators to subdivide the avoidant attachment category into dismissing avoidant and fearful avoidant groups, the former a defensive, denial-oriented style that is deadened to attachment and the latter a more vulnerable style that is fearful of emotional pain, but desirous of attachment. This differentiation of two types of avoidant attachment (dismissive and fearful) have been validated with independent assessments from peers, partners, and coworkers. In addition, the preoccupied attachment category can be similarly subdivided into subcategories of compulsive caregiving and compulsive careseeking, with the former being more developmentally advanced than the latter. These and other findings suggest that developmental levels can be distinguished within the internal working models of the various attachment categories and that these developmental distinctions have not yet been fully explored and articulated by attachment researchers and theorists.

For example, Levy and Blatt cite research which indicates that the variants of avoidant and preoccupied attachment categories identified with a self-report attachment instrument (BAQ), are associated with different developmental levels of self and object representations and with different ways of regulating affect. Fearful avoidant subjects tend to give more articulated and differentiated descriptions of self and significant others than do dismissing avoidant subjects, while compulsive caregivers tend to have more adaptive ways of regulating affect

than do compulsive careseekers. Integrating findings on the relationship of attachment status with type of depression, Levy and Blatt
conclude that "the variability in the level of integration and differentiation of mental representation within, as well as between, attachment
categories suggests that each category encompasses individuals with
different levels of object relations development and adaptive potentials." They conclude that the integration of cognitive developmental
and object relations perspectives with attachment theory refines and
enriches our understanding of internal working models and interpersonal behaviors that accompany the different attachment patterns.

In "The Two-Person Unconscious: Intersubjective Dialogue, Enactive Relational Representation, and the Emergence of New Forms of
Relational Organization," a paper that grew out of the Process of
Change Study Group of the Boston Psychoanalytic Institute, Karlen
Lyons-Ruth integrates the findings of attachment research with
findings from infant research on early intersubjective exchanges
between mother and infant by Stern, Trevarthan, and others to
advance a theory of therapeutic change. According to Lyons-Ruth,
attachment researchers have delineated the broad strokes of attachment organization, in both representational and behavioral aspects,
but we must turn to microanalytic research of the mother–infant interaction to develop a more finely nuanced picture of the enactive representational structures or procedural representations that underlie
attachment categories. Lyons-Ruth integrates the attachment concept
with the concept of intersubjectivity as developed by Stern (1985) and
others, arguing that maternal sensitivity, which has been hypothesized
by some to be the bedrock of secure attachment, is made up of micro-
moments of collaborative dialogue between parent and child involving
ongoing monitoring and empathic responsivity to the infant's subjective reality (which encompasses affectivity, intentionality, and cognition) out of which come procedural representations that are at the
bedrock of the attachment behavioral system. Lyons-Ruth states that
attachment research, most notably the accretion of evidence on the
ways in which parents unconsciously perpetuate their own attachment
histories in direct parent–infant transactions, has provided us with
powerful evidence for these early forms of procedural knowing or
memory—behavioral schemas that are expressed through repetition
and enactment, rather than through symbolic coding or lexical expres-

sion. Thus, Lyons-Ruth enlarges our understanding of the nature of internal working models of attachment, which she defines as enactive procedural representations of how to do things with others. These procedural representations are rooted in early parent–infant interactions, which are represented in enactive form, not only from the earliest months of life, but also as the individual matures.

Indeed, Lyons-Ruth argues that development does not inevitably move from the procedural to the symbolic memory, from primary to secondary process thought, or from enactive to lexical modes of representation, but that the procedural, enactive, primary mode persists as a vital force and motivator throughout development. These formulations are consistent with earlier revisions of psychoanalytic thought presented by Merton Gill (1976), Robert Holt (1967), and others. Lyons-Ruth hypothesizes that, while there is continual cross-referencing between the symbolic and the procedural and between enactive and lexical modes of representation, they each remain distinct ways of experiencing and being with self and others and that enactive relational knowing is infused with primary schemas and affects that may in fact exert a continual shaping influence on symbolic systems. Thus, she poses a challenge to the hegemony of the verbally mediated arena of symbolic communication between analyst and analysand and, instead, highlights the importance of procedural knowledge and enactive representations both in early development and in analytic exchanges.

Lyons-Ruth asserts that because relational meaning systems are encoded in the enactive or imagistic, rather than lexical, modes of representation and involve cognitive understanding as well as affective reciprocal exchanges, therapeutic change may occur in these various representational modalities. Some of these formulations are continuous with other points of view within psychoanalysis, including those of Blatt and Behrends (1987), Lichtenberg (1983), Loewald (1980), and Winnicott (1971) on the nature of therapeutic action. Lyons-Ruth demonstrates the importance of these formulations for attachment theory, but she calls for a major revision of psychoanalytic categories based on the above formulations. She argues, for example, that the most powerful aspect of therapeutic dialogue and therapeutic change may be represented in the enactive or procedural mode, which places reciprocal intersubjective exchanges, rather than interpretation, at the heart of psychoanalysis. Furthermore, in her view, the process of working through in psychoanalysis involves the development of new implicit procedures that better reflect and are adapted to current reality—a process that occurs primarily at the enactive level. Implicit knowledge about the relationship on the part of patient and therapist develops in tandem with, but is not reducible to, the unfolding of transference and countertransference dynamics. The centrality of implicit relational knowing for the intrapersonal and interpersonal worlds also has implications, according to Lyons-Ruth, for the theory of internalization, which she views as occurring at a presymbolic level. Indeed, for Lyons-Ruth, the primary form of representation is one of "implicit relational knowing," which is not translatable into symbolic modes of representation. These formulations represent another chapter in the long debate about the extent to which the development of a shared implicit relationship or the interpretation of transference and resistance constitute the primary mutative force in psychoanalysis (Loewald, 1980; Lichtenberg, 1983; Blatt and Behrends, 1987; Stern et al., 1998).

In the final paper in this issue, "The Development of Caregiving: A Comparison of Attachment Theory and Psychoanalytic Approaches to Mothering," Carol George and Judith Solomon integrate concepts from both attachment and psychoanalytic theory to develop a comprehensive model of the caregiving behavioral system—a model that not only integrates but also transcends the bounds of both theoretical traditions and, as such, provides an example of the type of creative thinking that can ensue when the traditions are used as springboards rather than strictures. The authors begin by comparing and contrasting psychoanalytic and attachment conceptualizations of caregiving. Theorists in both traditions highlight the significance of the mother's empathic responsivity to infant needs and cues for self-development and relatedness, the importance of the fundamental interconnection between mother and child for personality development, and the mother as catalyst for age-appropriate development. Both psychoanalysis and attachment theory have increasingly moved to the view that caregiving is a bidirectional process involving reciprocal behaviors between parent and child. Psychoanalytic thinkers have reached this conclusion through experiences in the consulting room and attachment theorists through systematic observation of mother-infant interaction.

Despite these areas of similarity, George and Solomon assert that an understanding of mothering from an attachment perspective as an independent, motivational behavioral system, one that is complementary with but distinct from the attachment behavioral system, provides an ethologically grounded view of caregiving that expands both attachment and psychoanalytic theory. In accordance with much recent attachment research, George and Solomon focus on the mother's representational processes and the meaning to her of becoming a caregiver for the child. The authors also emphasize that caregiving, as an independent motivational system, can come into conflict with other motivational systems, such as those that revolve around eros or work. While such an expanded view of motivation is not consistent with a classic psychoanalytic perspective that continues to give primary focus to the dual-drive theory, the idea of conflict devolving from the intersection of motivational forces is congruent with psychoanalytic views on the ubiquitous nature of conflict (Brenner, 1994). Furthermore, the view of caregiving as a developmental process that leads to an autonomous behavioral system that is distinct but synchronous with the infant's attachment behavioral system is firmly rooted in attachment theory, but owes much to psychoanalytic theory. The derivatives of the caregiving behavioral system are first evident as pretend maternal behaviors in toddlerhood, are consolidated in adolescence with hormonal and neurological changes that make childbearing possible, and come to fruition during the transition to parenthood—a transition with momentous psychological and physical aspects, including the hormonal, neurological, and psychological changes catalyzed by birth, parturition, and early mother–child closeness and bonding. Following previous psychoanalytic theorists such as Benedek (1959), George and Solomon suggest that the powerful dynamic experiences of parenthood may in fact lead parents to rework their own internalized experiences of parenting and bring about fundamental revisions of their own core mental representations.

Such a psychoanalytically informed developmental perspective on the evolution of caregiving, in turn, allows for fresh perspectives on the transgenerational transmission of caretaking patterns. Attachment investigators have identified the lawful predictability and evolution in patterns of attachment by empirically linking the parent's state of mind with regard to attachment as assessed on the Adult Attachment Interview (AAI) with the infant–parent behaviors observed in the Ainsworth Strange Situation (Main et al., 1985; Fonagy et al., 1991). However, attachment researchers have also concerned themselves with identifying the mechanisms of change from insecure to secure attachment status. George and Solomon hypothesize that the experiences of pregnancy and parturition in conjunction with the new attachment experiences provided by interactions with the infant, may catalyze such a shift to security in parents initially assessed in the prenatal period as having insecure states of mind regarding attachment. In support of this hypothesis on the experience of parenthood as a potential mechanism of change from insecure to secure states of mind regarding attachment, George and Solomon cite research studies which indicate that mothers whose state of mind regarding attachment was judged insecure during the prenatal period were more likely to have infants classified as secure than were parents judged secure in the prenatal period to have infants classified as insecure.

Joe Lichtenberg, who has been a rigorous advocate of the importance of attachment theory and research for psychoanalytic thought, provides an integrative discussion that in itself makes creative contributions to the topic at hand. In the context of a discussion that appreciates the unique contributions of each paper, Lichtenberg also identifies and addresses controversies that emerge from the dialogue in the papers between two theoretical systems which he maintains are mutually enriching but distinct. For example, Lichtenberg suggests that attachment theory, in emphasizing the survival value of the child's strategies to maintain proximity to the parent in the face of separation and loss, provided psychoanalytic object relations theory with a firm evolutionary basis. However, he hypothesizes that the proclivity toward intersubjective communication and toward affectionate exchanges, observed both in early development and in the consulting room, may have an independent evolutionary substrate (in that both affection and communication also insure proximity) that is not adequately accounted for by the attachment motivational concept. Lichtenberg calls for an expansion of the attachment construct to accommodate aspects of human symbolic communication and libidinal exchanges that are not fully represented under current conceptualization of the various patterns of secure and insecure attachment.

Not only does he highlight the aspects of these papers that are useful for the further development and amplification of both psycho-analytic and attachment theory, but he also translates those aspects of attachment theory and research addressed in the papers that are applicable to psychoanalytic practice. As in all good translations, the transposition of attachment concepts into the clinical realm involves a new creation that reflects but does not directly replicate the original source. Concepts of resistance and defense, for example, are reexamined by Lichtenberg in the light of the contributions of attachment theory and research. Narrative organizing patterns encompass pervasive attachment strategies that encompass but are not reducible to different defensive structures and therefore only partially amenable to defense interpretation. In addition, Lichtenberg suggests that, like diagnostic categories, the major attachment classifications and the further refinements of them reported in this issue provide an organizing framework for the practicing analyst, which expands our understanding of early relational procedures that may be reexperienced in the therapeutic arena. Although the attachment categories may amplify diagnostic understanding, the clinician in practice must remain attuned to the subtleties of transference manifestations, which may fleetingly take a secure, dismissing, preoccupied or unresolved (for trauma and loss) configuration depending not only on the patient's history, but on the current interactions with the analyst. In this regard, Lichtenberg invites analysts to assess attachment theory's utility according to their own clinical experience, thereby bringing to fruition Bowlby's dream that clinicians "test the theories use" (Bowlby, 1988, p. ix).

REFERENCES

Ainsworth, M. D. S., (1985), Patterns of mother infant attachments: antecedents and effects on development. *Bull. NY Acad. Med.,* 61:792–812.
———— Blehar, M.C., Waters, E. & Wall, S. (1978), *Patterns of Attachment.* Hillsdale, NJ: Lawrence Erlbaum.

———— Allen, J. P., Hauser, S. T. & Borman-Spurrell, E. (1996), Attachment theory as a framework for understanding sequelae of severe adolescent psychopathology: An eleven year follow-up study. *J. Consult. & Clin. Psychol.*, 61:254–253.

Balint, M. (1952), On love and hate. *Internat. J. Psycho-Anal.*, 33:355–362.

———— (1959), *Thrills and Regressions*. London: Hogarth Press.

Benedek, T. (1959), Parenthood as a developmental phase: A contribution to the libido theory. *J. Amer. Psychoanal. Assn.*, 7:389–417.

Bion, W. (1967), *Second Thoughts*. London: Heinemann.

Blatt, S. J. & Behrends (1987), Internalization, separation-individuation, and the nature of therapeutic actions. *Internat. J. Psycho-Anal.*, 68:279–297.

———— & Ford, R. Q. (1994), *Therapeutic Change*. New York: Plenum.

———— & Homann, E. (1992), Parent–child interaction in the etiology of dependent and self-critical depression. *Clin. Psychol. Rev.*, 12:47–91.

———— Stayner, D. A., Auerbach, J. S. & Behrends, R. S. (1996), Change in object and self representations in long-term intensive inpatient treatment of seriously disturbed adolescents and young adults. *Psychiatry*, 59:82–107.

Bowlby, J. (1958), The nature of the child's tie to his mother. *Internat. J. Psycho-Anal.*, 39:350–373.

———— (1969), *Attachment and Loss. Vol. 1: Attachment*. New York: Basic Books, 1982.

———— (1973), *Attachment and Loss. Vol. 2: Separation*. New York: Basic Books.

———— (1977), The making and breaking of affectional bonds. I. Aetiology and psychopathology in the light of attachment theory. *Brit. J. Psychiat.*, 130:201–210.

———— (1978), *Attachment Theory and Its Therapeutic Implications*. Chicago: University of Chicago Press.

———— (1980), *Attachment and Loss. Vol. 3: Loss, Sadness and Depression*. New York: Basic Books.

———— (1988), *A Secure Base*. New York: Basic Books.

Brenner, C. (1994), The mind as conflict and compromise formation. *J. Clin. Psychoanal.*, 3:473–488.

Cassidy, J. (1994), Emotion regulation: Influences of attachment relationships. *Monog. Soc. Research Child Devel.*, 59:53–72 (Serial No. 240).

———— (1995), Attachment and generalized anxiety disorder. In: *Emotion, Cognition and Representation*, ed. D. Cicchetti & S. Toth. New York: Wiley, pp. 343–369.

Cicchetti, D. & Cohen, D. J. (1995), *Developmental Psychopathology: Risk, Disorder and Adaptation, Vol. 2*. New York: Wiley.

Diamond, D. & Blatt, S. J. (1994), Internal working models of attachment and psychoanalytic theories of the representational world: A comparison and critique. In: *Attachment in Adults*, M. B. Sperling & W. H. Berman. New York: Guilford Press, pp. 72–97.

Dozier, M. (1990), Attachment organization and treatment use for adults with serious psychopathological disorders. *Dev. & Psychopathol.*, 2:47–60.

———— Cue, K. & Barnett, L. (1993), Clinicians as caregivers: Role of attachment organization in treatment. *J. Consult. & Clin. Psychol.*, 62:793–800.

Fairbairn, W. R. D. (1952), *An Object-Relations Theory of the Personality*. New York: Basic Books.

Farber, B. A., Lippert, R. A. & Nevas, D. B. (1995), The therapist as attachment figure. *Psychotherapy*, 32:204–212.

Fonagy, P. (1991), Thinking about thinking. *Internat. J. Psycho-Anal.*, 72:639–656.

――― (1998), Moments of change in psychoanalytic theory: Discussion of a new theory of psychic change. *Inf. Mental H. J.*, 19:346–353.

――― Steele, H. & Steele, M. (1991), Maternal representations of attachment during pregnancy predict the organization of infant–mother attachment at one year of age. *Child Devel.*, 62:891–905.

――― Steele, M., Steele, H., Leigh, T., Kennedy, R., Mattoon, G. & Target, M. (1995), Attachment, the reflective self and borderline states: The predictive specificity of the Adult Attachment Interview and pathological emotional development. In: *Attachment Theory: Social, Developmental and Clinical Perspectives*, ed. S. Goldberg, R. Muir & J. Kerr. Hillsdale, NJ: The Analytic Press, pp. 233–279.

――― Leigh, T., Steele, M., Steele, H., Kennedy, R., Mattoon, G., Target, M. & Gerber, A. (1996), The relation of attachment status, psychiatric classification and response to psychotherapy. *J. Consult. & Clin. Psychol.*, 64:22–31.

George, C. O., Kaplan, N. & Main, M. (1985), The Berkeley Adult Attachment Interview. Unpublished manuscript, Department of Psychology, University of California, Berkeley.

Gill, M. M. (1976), Metapsychology is not psychology. In: *Psychology Versus Metapsychology*, ed. M. M. Gill & P. S. Holzman. New York: International Universities Press, pp. 71–105.

Hamilton, V. (1987), Some problems in the clinical application of attachment theory. *Psychoanal. Psychother.*, 3:67–83.

Hanly, M. Γ. (1996), Narrative now and then: A critical realist approach. *Internat. J. Psycho-Anal.*, 77:445–457.

Hartmann, H. (1958), *Ego Psychology and the Problem of Adaptation* (trans. D. Rapaport). New York: International Universities Press.

Hesse, E. (1996), Discourse, memory and the Adult Attachment Interview: A note with emphasis on the emerging Cannot Classify Category. *Inf. Mental Hlth. J.*, 17:4–11.

――― (1999), The adult attachment interview. In: *Handbook of Attachment*, ed. J. Cassidy & P. R. Shaver. New York: Guilford Press.

Holmes, J. (1993a), Attachment theory: A biological basis for psychotherapy. *Brit. J. Psychiat.*, 163:430–438.

――― (1993b), *John Bowlby and Attachment Theory*. London: Routledge.

――― (1995), Something there is that doesn't love a wall: John Bowlby, attachment theory and psychoanalysis. In: *Attachment Theory: Social, Developmental, and Clinical Perspectives*, ed. S. Goldberg, R. Muir & J. Kerr. Hillsdale, NJ: The Analytic Press, pp. 19–43.

――― (1996), *Attachment, Intimacy and Autonomy*. Northvale, NJ: Aronson.

Holt, R. R. (1967), The development of the primary process: A Structural view. In: *Motives and Thought*, ed. R. R. Holt. New York: International Universities Press, pp. 345–383.

Kernberg, O. (1975), *Borderline Conditions and Pathological Narcissism*. New York: Aronson.

――― (1990), New perspectives in psychoanalytic affect theory. In *Emotion: Theory, Research and Experience, Vol. 5*. New York: Academic Press.

Klein, M. (1935), A contribution to the psychogenesis of manic-depressive states. In: *Love, Guilt and Reparation & Other Works 1921–1945*. New York: Dell, 1975.

――― (1946), Notes on some schizoid mechanisms. In: *Envy and Gratitude and Other Works 1946–1963*. New York: Dell, 1975.

Lichtenberg, J. (1983), *Psychoanalysis and Infant Research*. Hillsdale, NJ: The Analytic Press.

———— (1992), *Psychoanalysis and Motivation*. Hillsdale, NJ: The Analytic Press.

Liotti, G. (1995), Disorganized/disoriented attachment in the psychotherapy of the dissociative disorders. In: *Attachment Theory: Social, Developmental and Clinical Perspectives*, ed. S. Goldberg, R. Muir, & J. Kerr. Hillsdale, NJ: The Analytic Press, pp. 343–367.

Loewald, H. W. (1980), The therapeutic action of psychoanalysis. In: *Papers on Psychoanalysis*. New Haven: Yale University Press.

Luthar, S. S., Burack, J. & Cicchetti, D., eds. (1997), *Developmental Psychopathology*. London: Cambridge University Press.

Mahler, M. S., Pine, F. & Bergman, A. (1975), *The Psychological Birth of the Human Infant*. New York: Basic Books.

Main, M. (1991), Metacognitive knowledge, metacognitive monitoring, and singular (coherent) vs. multiple (incoherent) models of attachment: Findings and directions for future research. In: *Attachment Across the Life Cycle*, ed. C. M. Parkes, J. Stevenson-Hinde & P. Marris. London: Routledge, pp. 127–159.

———— (1995), Attachment: Overview, with implications for clinical work. In: *Attachment Theory: Social, Developmental and Clinical Perspectives*. ed. S. Goldberg, R. Muir & J. Kerr. Hillsdale, NJ: The Analytic Press, pp. 233–279.

———— (1999), Epilogue. Attachment Theory: Eighteen points with suggestions for future studies. In: *Handbook of Attachment*, ed. J. Cassidy & P. R. Shaver. New York: Guilford Press.

———— & Goldwyn, R. (1994), Adult attachment scoring and classification system. Unpublished scoring manual. Department of Psychology, University of California, Berkeley.

———— & Morgan, H. (1996), Disorganization and disorientation in infant strange situation behavior: Phenotypic resemblance to dissociative states. In: *Handbook of Dissociation*, ed. L. K. Michelson & W. J. Ray. New York: Plenum Press. pp. 107–137.

———— Kaplan, N., & Cassidy, J. (1985), Security in infancy, childhood, and adulthood: A move to the level of representation. In: *Monog. Soc. Research Child Devel.*, Chicago: University of Chicago Press, 209:66–104.

Patrick, M., Hobson, R.P., Castle, D., Howard, R. & Maughn, B. (1994), Personality disorder and the mental representation of early social experience. *Devel. & Psychopathol.*, 6:375–388.

Schafer, R. (1992), *Retelling a Life*. New York: Basic Books.

Silverman, D. (1991), Attachment patterns and Freudian theory: An integrative proposal. *Psychoanal. Psychol.*, 8:169–193.

———— (1994), Attachment research: An approach to a developmental relational perspective. In: *Relational Perspectives in Psychoanalysis*, ed. N. J. Skolnick & S. O. Warshaw. Hilldale, NJ: The Analytic Press, pp. 195–216.

———— (1998), The tie that binds: Affect regulation, attachment and psychoanalysis. *Psychoanul. Psychol.*, 15:187–212.

Slade, A., (1999), Attachment Theory and research. Implications for theory and practice of individual psychotherapy. In: *Handbook of Attachment Theory and Research*, ed. J. Cassidy & P. Shaver. New York: Guilford Press.

———— & Aber, J. L. (1992), Attachments, drives, and development: Conflicts and convergences in theory. In: *The Interface of Psychoanalysis and Psychology*, ed. J.

Barron, M. Eagle, & D. Wolitsky. Washington, D.C.: American Psychological Association, pp. 154–185.

Stern, D. (1985), *The Interpersonal World of the Infant*. New York: Basic Books.

———— Sander, L. W., Nahum, J. P., Harrison, A. M., Lyons-Ruth, K., Morgan, A., Bruschweiler-Stern, N. & Tronick, E. Z. (1998), Non-interpretive mechanisms in psychoanalytic therapy: The "something more" than interpretation. *Internat. J. Psycho-Anal.*, 79:902–921.

Wallerstein, R. S. (1986), *Forty-two Lives in Treatment*. New York: Guilford Press.

———— (1988), Assessment of structural change in psychoanalytic therapy and research. J. Amer. Psychoanal. Assn. 36 (suppl): 241–261.

Weston, D. (1997), Towards a clinically and empirically sound theory of motivation. *Internat. J. Psycho-Anal.*, 78:521–548.

Winnicott, D. W. (1960), Ego distortion in terms of true and false self. In: *The Maturational Processes and the Facilitating Environment*. London: Hogarth Press, 1965, pp. 140–152.

———— (1971), Transitional objects and transitional phenomena. In: *Playing and Reality*. Middlesex, UK: Penguin Books, pp. 1–30.

Diana Diamond, Ph.D.
Sidney J. Blatt, Ph.D.
Issue Editors

Points of Contact and Divergence Between Psychoanalytic and Attachment Theories: Is Psychoanalytic Theory Truly Different

PETER FONAGY, Ph.D., FBA

IT IS GENERALLY ACCEPTED BY PSYCHOANALYSTS that there is something wrong with attachment theory. Following the publication of John Bowlby's paper in *The Psychoanalytic Study of the Child* (Bowlby, 1960), leading psychoanalytic developmentalists were quick to point to the limitations of attachment theory—its mechanistic, nondynamic quality, and its misrepresentation of psychoanalytic ideas (A. Freud, 1960; Schur, 1960; Spitz, 1960). Opposition to attachment theory for once united the warring factions of the British Psycho-Analytical Society (the Anna Freudians and the Kleinians) (Grosskruth, 1986). Many major figures contributed to this one-sided debate between psychoanalysis and attachment theory (e.g., Engel, 1971; Rochlin, 1971; Kernberg, 1976a; Roiphe, 1976; Hanly, 1978).

Their critiques, while complex and scholarly, could be summarized under relatively few headings: (1) Attachment theory simplifies out of existence the unconscious motivational system that is considered to underpin behavior (drives, the system unconscious, and complex internalized motivational and conflict-resolving systems depicted, for example, in the structural model). (2) Attachment theory excludes from consideration the richness and diversity of human affect states

Dr. Fonagy is Freud Memorial Professor of Psychoanalysis, University College London; Director of Research, The Anna Freud Centre, and Director, Child and Family Center and Center for Outcomes Research and Effectiveness, Menninger Foundation.

(e.g., signal affects experienced by the ego, the socialization of pleasures from the infant's physical body). (3) Attachment theory ignores biological vulnerabilities of the infant other than those rooted in caregiver behavior, and even here it is severely restricted to experiences of neglect or separation. (4) Attachment theory ignores psychoanalytic discoveries concerning the development of the ego, particularly developments beyond infancy (e.g., during the anal and oedipal phases), even when considering its paradigmatic dyadic construct: separation and loss. (5) Attachment theory fails to consider aspects of the child–parent relationship that are not rooted in experiences of separation, for example, aspects that are the products of projection, primitive internalizations. (6) Attachment theory is reductionist in stressing evolutionary considerations at the expense of the full recognition of complex human symbolic functioning. The common theme here is that attachment theory, by adopting the criterion of operationalizability for admissible theoretical constructs, drastically reduces the explanatory power of psychoanalytic observations.

Attachment theorists could take issue with each and every one of these points. For example, Bretherton's work on internal working models belies the assertion that internal, symbolic processes are ignored or underemphasized in attachment theory (Bretherton, 1987, 1995). Kernberg (1976a) directly took issue with Bowlby for not taking account of "the internal world" and for neglecting "instinct as intra-psychic development and internalised object relations as major structural organisers of psychic reality" (p. 121). This was undoubtedly an unwarranted criticism, particularly in the light of Bowlby's emphasis on constructs such as the internal working model (Bowlby, 1969, chapter 17). It might have been more accurate to say that Bowlby's conceptualization of the internal world was different from Kernberg's. Kernberg made no reference to Bowlby's later book (Bowlby, 1973) and was also silent on Bowlby's restatement of the psychoanalytic concept of the internal world in terms of "environmental and organismic models" (Bowlby, 1969, p. 82). By and large, the psychoanalytic critique of attachment theory is outdated, based on misapprehension, and is poorly informed about the empirical and clinical observations that this body of ideas has generated.

These qualifications can equally well be applied to attachment theory representations of psychoanalytic ideas. Bowlby maintained a

blinkered attitude to psychoanalysis. Perhaps sensitized by psychoanalytic critiques of attachment theory, he offered generalizations of the
psychoanalytic model which bear the hallmarks of straw figures (e.g.,
Bowlby, 1973, chapter 22; 1980b, p. 310). Thus, just as psychoanalysts tend to misread attachment theory and find it wanting in depth
and explanatory power, so Bowlby and other attachment theorists
selectively focus on the weakest aspects of the psychoanalytic corpus.
Both sides appear to be determined to forestall the possibility of a
mutually clarifying interaction. There are major figures who have
consistently bucked this trend (Bretherton, 1987; Lichtenberg, 1989;
Holmes, 1993, 1997; Eagle, 1995, 1997; Shane, Shane, and Gales,
1997). Nevertheless, a more balanced reconsideration of the interrela-
tionship of these two substantive bodies of theoretical ideas seems
timely. In this paper I will attempt to identify a common core to
psychoanalytic and attachment theory and then go on to elaborate
areas where attachment theory could particularly benefit from greater
psychoanalytic sophistication. It is beyond the scope of this paper to
consider the ways in which psychoanalytic clinical or theoretical work
could gain from closer contact with attachment theory.

What Is There in Common Between
Psychoanalytic Theories and Attachment Theory?

Since psychoanalytic theory cannot, at its current stage of evolution,
be reduced to a singular coherent set of propositions, points of contact
can only be identified between attachment theory and particular traditions of psychoanalytic thought. The points of contact listed below are
not meant to be exhaustive or even representative, merely illustrative—arguments to put to rest the prevailing view of incompatibility
between these two frames of reference.

(1) Personality Development Is Best Studied in Relation
to the Child's Social Environment

Freud (1954) and Bowlby (1946) both began their theoretical contributions with concern about the psychological consequences of early
deprivation. Freud's celebrated turning away from the "seduction
hypothesis" (Masson, 1984) did not compromise his position on the

pathogenesis of childhood trauma (Freud, 1917, p. 370; 1931, p. 232; 1939, pp. 75–76). Modern psychoanalytic readers might criticize Bowlby for the therapeutic realism of his approach and his emphasis on the therapeutic qualities of cathartic recollections of traumatic events (Bowlby, 1977). However, far from going back to the naïve realism of Freud's early theories, Bowlby's attention to the representation of experience (Bowlby, 1980a) represents an elaboration of the fourth phase of Freud's theory, the structural model (Freud, 1923). Freud, in common with Bowlby, recognized that anxiety was a biologically determined epiphenomenal experience linked to the perception of both external and internal dangers (Freud, 1926), the psychological template for which was loss of the object. The move towards recognizing that adaptation to the external world had to be an essential component of the psychoanalytic account and that such an account necessitated a reorganization of the theory in terms of a quasicognitive structure (Schafer, 1983) is the essential common background for both ego psychological and attachment theory elaborations of the classical psychoanalytical model.

Bowlby was not the first psychoanalyst to focus on interpersonal, rather than intrapsychic, factors in pathogenesis. The Hungarian psychoanalyst Ferenczi (1933) pointed to the potentially traumatic nature of the adult's failure to understand meanings in the child's psychological world, thus anticipating risks associated with lack of sensitivity on the part of the child's primary objects. The emphasis on the quality of caregiving has run through most of the dominant psychoanalytic traditions since Ferenczi, but it played a particularly dominant role in the work of Spitz (1945, 1965), Erickson (1950, 1959), Winnicott (1962), and Anna Freud (1941–1945, 1955). Is there an underlying epistemic difference then between how psychoanalysts and attachment theorists conceptualize the influence of the social environment? In fact, these views have much in common:

(1) *Actual versus psychic reality:* It is a fundamental tenet of both theories that social perception and social experience are distorted by expectations, both conscious and unconscious. Freud's description in the structural model (Freud, 1923) of the ego's capacity to create defenses that organize characterological and symptomatic constructions as part of the

developmental process became a cornerstone of Bowlby's trilogy, particularly the last volume (Bowlby, 1980a). Anna Freud's description of common mechanisms of defense (Freud, 1936) can be readily restated in terms of mental representation or, rather, its typical distortions (Sandler and Rosenblatt, 1962; Sandler, 1987a). Crittenden's (1990) work has been particularly helpful in translating behaviors typical of avoidant and resistant attachment patterns into the language of the defensive behaviors of infancy (Fraiberg, 1982). More recently, we have attempted to demonstrate that transgenerational consistencies in attachment classification may be understood as internalization of the caregiver's defenses mobilized by the infant's distress (Fonagy et al., 1995a). Thus both attachment theory and modern psychoanalysis have as their fundamental epistemic aim the description of the internal mechanisms responsible for the discrepancy between actual and psychic reality.

(2) *Emphasis on early life:* It hardly needs demonstrating that both psychoanalysts and attachment theorists privilege the first years of life in their consideration of the relationship between social environment and personality development. Within psychoanalysis, this bias took some years to fully emerge and did so more or less contemporaneously with the development of Bowlby's ideas. For some time Melanie Klein's attempts to consider the first year of life as setting a template for subsequent phases of personality development (Klein, 1935) were treated with skepticism by psychoanalytic developmentalists, particularly because of the level of cognitive sophistication she appeared to be willing to attribute to the infant in the first year of life (Yorke, 1971). More sophisticated methods of observations of infant behavior, however, revealed the human infant to possess relatively complex mental capacities, even at birth, in some cases exceeding that which was presupposed by Kleinian theory (Gergely, 1992). Margaret Mahler is commonly credited with bringing observational methods to bear on the earliest phases of development. Her systematic observational studies, however, were based upon children in their third year of life (Gergely,

submitted). In fact, much of the later criticism of Mahler's theories (e.g., Klein, 1981; Stern, 1985) focuses upon the fact that her characterizations of the earliest phases of the psychological birth of the infant are based on retrospective pathomorphic extrapolations from adult mental disorders. The emergence of self psychology as an alternative psychoanalytic framework (Kohut, 1971) has contributed further to placing the earliest phases of development in the center of psychoanalytic theoretical interest. As concern with the real, as opposed to the reconstructed, infant grew within psychoanalysis, so did psychoanalytic interest increase in attachment theory (e.g., Lichtenberg, 1995).

(3) *Maternal sensitivity and mirroring:* Beyond sharing a converging interest in the early stages of development, there is a more specific common focus on maternal sensitivity as a causal factor in determining the quality of object relationships and therefore psychic development. However, the way in which the construct of maternal sensitivity is conceptualized is significantly different between attachment theory and psychoanalytic theory of development. Attachment theory describes sensitivity in a variety of ways that all involve behavior or personality characteristics of the caregiver (e.g., global ratings of responsiveness, accuracy of individual responses, personality traits of the caregiver, the quality of mental representation of the infant in the caregiver's mind) (De Wolff and van IJzendoorn, 1997). In psychoanalytic formulations sensitivity tends to be considered in terms of its consequences, its organizing impact on the child's self-development. There is also considerable heterogeneity among these conceptualizations. The Kleinian formulation of sensitive caregiving would be of a parent capable of absorbing and retransmitting the infant's psychological experience in a "metabolized" form (Bion, 1967). The infant can accept and reinternalize what had been projected and transformed, thus creating a representation of these internal moments of interaction with the caretaker that it can tolerate. In time, Bion suggested, infants internalize the function of transformation and will acquire the capacity to regulate their own negative

affective states. The nonverbal nature of this process implies that physical proximity of the caregiver is essential. Thus Bion's ideas may provide us with an alternative perspective of the sociobiological root of the infant's need for proximity to the psychological caregiver, the adult mind.

In a slightly different vein, Winnicott (1956) proposed that, when the baby looks at the mother, who is reflecting the baby's state, what he apprehends in the mother's expression is his own self-state. Thus the mother's mirroring function is seen as essential for the establishment of the baby's self-representation. In Kohut's work (1971, 1977), probably as a consequence of his clinical interest in narcissism, the empathy concept was closely tied to considerations of self-evaluation (self-esteem). The psychoanalyst whose formulation most closely matches attachment theory concerns with caregiver behavior was Erik Erikson (1950). Erikson (1964), for example, conceived of basic trust as arising out of "the experience of the caretaking person as a *coherent* being, who reciprocates one's physical and emotional needs and therefore deserves to be endowed with trust, and whose face is recognised as it recognises" (p. 117).

There is further indication that psychoanalytic concepts of sensitivity and those of attachment theorists pertain to related phenomena. Both attachment theorists and psychoanalysts have come to the conclusion that the ideal level of caregiver sensitivity from the point of view of infant development is moderate rather than perfect, both in terms of intensity and responsibility for the infant's state. Certainly, this idea is at the heart of Winnicott's notion of "good enough" parenting (Winnicott, 1962), Kohut's model of transmuting internalization (Kohut and Wolf, 1978) and, most explicitly, Erikson's writings. In *Childhood and Society* (1950) he writes: "A certain ratio between the positive and the negative, which if the balance is towards the positive, will help him to meet later crises with a better chance of unimpaired development" (p. 61). Erikson saw nonintrusiveness of the parent (Malatesta et al., 1986) as the mother not trying to control the interaction too much. Interactional synchrony (Isabella and Belsky, 1991) is probably equivalent to Erikson's description of "reciprocity or mutual regulation." There is a shared common assumption that a well-regulated relationship with the caregiver leads to an autonomous, robust sense of self. Thus while attachment theory and psychoanalytic formulations certainly differ in terms of their respective emphasis on caregiver behavior versus infant experience, in neither domain has a definitive formulation as yet emerged. We will suggest later that this critical facet of social development for both theories may provide an important area of cross-fertilization.

(4) *The motivation for forming relationships:* Contrary to Bowlby's prejudiced claims, modern psychoanalysis shares the fundamental assumption of attachment theory that the infant–caregiver relationship is not based on physical need but rather on some kind of independent autonomous need for a relationship. Bowlby's motivation to assert divergence from psychoanalysis on this point (Bowlby, 1958) may have in part been rhetorical; after all, as with any new theory in this field, new ideas stand out in greatest relief with the assertion of a dichotomy—even if this represents an oversimplification. More importantly, there is a lack of clarity arising out of overwhelming heterogeneity in psychoanalytic formulations on this point. Arnold Modell (1975), for example, suggested the existence of object relations instincts characterized by interaction processes rather than discharge. In the work of the British Object Relations School, the need for relationships is considered as a constitutional predisposition, which is described variously as "primary love" (Balint, 1952), "object seeking" (Fairbairn, 1952), "ego relatedness" (Winnicott, 1965), or "just personal relations" (Guntrip, 1961). Bowlby in certain places was explicit in his acknowledgment of these analysts but felt he went beyond them by establishing a firm biological and evolutionary basis for their constructs.

Even within the British school, however, there is ambiguity in the treatment of the relationship construct. While for Balint and Winnicott the construct is unequivocally primary, for Fairbairn and Guntrip, it is described as a need secondary to a primal need for psychic organization. This latter view is also

implicit in Kernberg's model, which suggests that the self
evolves as part of a relationship (1976a, 1976b), as a product
of internalization (introjection, identification, and ego
identity). Yet other psychoanalytic writers appear to assume
that the need for relationships arises as a defense against the
vicissitudes of the child's internal world. We have already
seen how the concept of proximity seeking may be derived
from Bion's notion of containment (Bion, 1967). Eric
Erikson's closeness to the drive theory tradition may have
also led him to infer that attachment played a secondary role,
either facilitating identity development or being its by-prod-
uct; it has the status of an intermediary link in the process of
development towards individuation (Erikson, 1968). In
summary, modern psychoanalysis does not differ from
attachment theory in the sense that it overlooks the child's
need for a relationship. There are, however, too many
competing formulations regarding the nature and origin of this
need. Thus the relevance of a singular and coherent account
drawn from attachment theory should be evident. This kind of
argument is beyond the scope of this paper.

(2) The Cognitive Underpinnings of Emotional Development

A major strength of attachment theory is the relative clarity with
which Bowlby describes the representational system, which mediates
and ensures the continuity of interpersonal behavior (Bowlby, 1969,
chapter 17). Bowlby's model has been elaborated and developed by
two pioneers in the field: Inge Bretherton (1987) and Mary Main
(Main, Kaplan, and Cassidy, 1985). Notwithstanding these advances,
there are many critics of the internal working models concept, particularly from among developmental psychologists (e.g., Dunn, 1996). At
the heart of such critiques is the lack of specificity of Bowlby's
model How do expectations concerning the likely response of a caregiver to the infant's distress develop into generalized templates for
social interaction? Mary Main's work on adults' discourse concerning
early relationships demonstrated suggestive links between infant
behavior in the strange situation and adult conversational styles—

manner of speech rather than narrative content (Main and Goldwyn, in preparation). Thus attachment theory and research have increasingly focused on procedural as opposed to episodic or semantic, memory systems (Schacter, 1992) in understanding the continuity of social behavior from infancy to adulthood. A case could be made that a similar family of ideas is emerging in the field of psychoanalysis. There are several issues of relevance:

(1) *The representation of relationships:* Originating in the work of Edith Jacobson (1954) it is now generally accepted that mental representations of relationships of self and object are key determinants of interpersonal behavior. She introduced the concept of representation to stress that these referred to the experiential impact of internal and external worlds and were subject to distortion and modification, irrespective of physical reality. A number of theorists have elaborated these notions in postulating that roles are encoded for both subject and objects. For example, Sandler (1976, 1987b) elaborated a model of the two-person interaction when the direct influence of one on the other is accounted for by the evocation of particular roles in the mind of the person who is being influenced. The behavior of the influencing person is seen as critical in eliciting a complementary response from the participant. Sandler suggests that in this way infantile patterns of relationships may be actualized or enacted in adult relationships. Daniel Stern (1994) and his coworkers in the Boston Psychoanalytic Institute (e.g., Morgan, 1998; Sander, in press; Stern, 1998; Tronick, 1998) have gone a step further in developing the idea that therapeutic change occurs, not as a consequence of insight or reflection on episodic memory, but as a consequence of experiences that change procedural (implicit) memory. Stern discusses the schemata of ways-of-being-with as an emergent property of the nervous system, which naturally aggregate the invariant aspects of interpersonal experience. He suggests (Stern, 1998) that these are the building blocks of internal working models, and while this remains to be demonstrated, his work suggests a route whereby the micro-experiences of infant–mother interaction

could become aggregated into enduring structures and subserve stable patterns of behavior.

(2) *The relationship context of cognitive development:* Both attachment theory and psychoanalytic theory assume that early relationships provide the context within which certain critical psychological functions are acquired and developed. Alan Sroufe (1990) offered an imaginative framework whereby early interaction patterns between infant and caregiver were thought to translate into individual styles for the regulation of affect, which in their turn determined patterns of interaction. Affect regulation is seen as internalized in the course of infant–caregiver interaction. Bretherton et al. (1979) and Main (1991) claim that the development of symbolic function is crucially dependent on the harmony of mother–infant interaction. These workers suggest that secure attachment frees attentional resources necessary for the full development of symbolic cognitive capacities.

The notion that psychic functions may be internalized from primary object relationships is present in the writings of a number of psychoanalytic authors. Rene Spitz (1945), in particular, saw the child's human partner as quickening the development of his innate abilities and mediating all perception, behavior, and knowledge. Spitz made specific reference to the role of mother–infant interaction in the development of self-regulation (see also Greenacre, 1952; Spitz, 1959). Bion's model of containment (Bion, 1959, 1962a) also assumes that the infant internalizes the function of transformation exercised by the caregiver and through this acquires the capacity to contain or regulate his own negative affective states. Winnicott (1953) makes a strong claim concerning the evolution of symbolic function in the "transitional space" between infant and caregiver. Winnicott bases this assertion on an assumption that three conditions pertain: (i) a sense of safety associated with experiencing the inner world, (ii) an opportunity for the infant deliberately to limit concern with external events, and (iii) an opportunity to generate spontaneous creative gestures. These parameters may be considered analogous to Bowlby's (1969) secure base notion. Both see the evolution of cognitive structure as a function of infant–mother interaction.

(3) *Mentalization in attachment theory and psychoanalysis:* A specific symbolic function that is central to both psychoanalytic and attachment theory and that emerged concurrently in psychoanalytic and attachment theory thinking is that of mentalization. Developmentalists over the past 10 years have drawn our attention to the universal and remarkable capacity of young children to interpret the behavior of themselves, as well as others, in terms of putative mental states (e.g., Morton and Frith, 1995). Reflective function enables children to conceive of others' beliefs, feelings, attitudes, desires, hopes, knowledge, imagination, pretense, plans, and so on. At the same time as making others' behavior meaningful and predictable, they are also able to activate flexibly from multiple sets of self–other representations the one most appropriate in a particular interpersonal context. Exploring the meaning of actions of others is crucially linked to the child's ability to label and find meaningful his or her own experience. This ability may make a critical contribution to affect regulation, impulse control, self-monitoring, and the experience of self-agency (Fonagy and Target, 1997).

Reflective function is closely linked to attachment. The frequency of both prospective mothers' and fathers' references to mental states in their accounts of their own childhood attachment experiences powerfully predicts the likelihood of their children being securely attached to them (Fonagy et al., 1991). If secure attachment is conceived of as the acquisition of procedures (implicit memories) for the regulation of aversive states of arousal (Cassidy, 1994; Carlsson and Sroufe, 1995; Sroufe, 1996), it may be argued that such information is most likely to be consistently acquired and coherently represented when the child's acute affective state is accurately, but not overwhelmingly, reflected back to the child. Secure attachment may thus have a great deal in common with successful containment (Bion, 1962a). Critical is the mother's mental capacity to contain the baby and respond, in terms of physical care, in a manner that shows awareness of the child's mental state yet reflect coping (mirroring distress while communicating an incompatible affect) (Fonagy et al., 1995b). If secure attachment is the product of successful containment, insecure attachment may be seen as the infant's identification with the caregiver's defensive behavior. A dismissing caregiver may fail to mirror the child's distress, while a preoccupied caregiver may represent the infant's state with excessive clarity. In either case, the opportunity for the child to internalize a representation of his mental state is lost. Proximity to the caregiver is in this case maintained at the cost of a compromise to reflective function.

Bowlby (1969) recognized the significance of the developmental step entailed in the emergence of "the child's capacity both to conceive of his mother as having her own goals and interests separate from his own and to take them into account" (p. 368). A number of empirical findings speak to the relationship of attachment security and reflective function. Attachment security is a good predictor of metacognitive capacity in the domains of memory, comprehension, and communication (Moss, Parent, and Gosselin, 1995). Attachment security with the mother has been found to be a good predictor of belief-desire reasoning in 3½- to 6-year-old children in both cross-sectional (Fonagy, Redfern, and Charman, 1997a) and longitudinal studies (Fonagy et al., submitted; Meins and Russell, 1997). On the basis of such findings, we have argued that the child's acquisition of reflective function, the tendency to incorporate mental state attributions into internal working models of self–other relationships, depends on the opportunities that he had in early life to observe and explore the mind of his primary caregiver. The parent of the secure child engages in behaviors such as pretend play, which almost obliges the child to contemplate the existence of mental states.

The caregiver's understanding of the child's mind encourages secure attachment; the caregiver's accurate reading of the child's mental state, moderated by indications that the adult has coped with the child's distress, underpins the symbolization of the internal state, which in turn leads to superior affect regulation (Gergely and Watson, 1996). Secure attachment provides a relatively firm base for the acquisition of a full understanding of minds. The secure infant feels safe in thinking about the mental state of the caregiver. By contrast, the avoidant child shuns the mental state of the other, while the resistant child focuses on its own state of distress to the exclusion of intersubjective exchanges. Disorganized infants may represent a separate category; hypervigilant to the caregiver's behavior, they may appear to be acutely sensitive to the caregiver's mental state yet fail to generalize this to their own mental state (self-organization) which remains disregulated and incoherent.

Is this model, derived from attachment theory, any different from traditional psychoanalytic accounts? We would argue "no" on a number of grounds. (1) The notion of reflective function or mentalization is already present in Freud's (1911) notion of *Bindung*, or linking. *Bindung* refers to the qualitative change from the physical (immediate) to the psychological (associative) quality of linking. (2) Melanie Klein (1945), in describing the depressive position, stressed that it necessarily entailed the recognition of hurt and suffering in the other, that is, the awareness of mental states. Although her emphasis is upon individual recognition of a destructive wish, clearly, this cannot arise without awareness of intentionality in both self and other. (3) We have already touched on Bion's (1962a, b) description of containment. He delineates the transformation ("alpha function") of internal events experienced as concrete ("beta elements") into tolerable, thinkable experiences. (4) Winnicott (1962) was perhaps closest to these ideas from attachment theory in recognizing the importance of the caregiver's *psychological* understanding of the infant in the emergence of the true self and in acknowledging the dialectical aspect of this relationship: The psychological self develops through perception of oneself in another person's mind as thinking and feeling. Parents who cannot reflect with understanding on their child's inner experience and respond accordingly deprive the child of a core psychological structure that he or she needs to build a viable sense of self. (5) Independently, French psychoanalysts developed a notion of mentalization, largely rooted in the economic point of view. Marty (1968) considered mentalization to be a protective buffer in the system preconscious with a capacity to prevent progressive disorganization. He saw mentalization as the function that linked drive excitations and internal representations and thereby created flexibility (both "fluidity" and "constancy") (Marty, 1990, 1991). Thus, according to Marty, mentalization ensures freedom in the use of associations, as well as permanence and stability, a description strikingly similar to Bowlby's account of the capacities of the securely attached child. (6) Another

French psychoanalyst, Pierre Luquet (1981, 1988), discussed the development of different forms of thinking and the reorganization of inner experience alongside this development. In his chapter on the theory of language (Luquet, 1987) he distinguished primary mental-ization (which is really the absence of mentalization or reflective capacity) from secondary (symbolic) mentalization. While this form of mentalization was still seen as closely connected to sensory data and primary unconscious fantasy, it was also seen as representative of these processes and observable in dreams, art, and play (see also Bucci, 1997). His third level was verbal thought, which he considered the most distant from bodily processes. Similar distinctions have been proposed by Green (1975), Segal (1957), McDougall (1978), and more recently in the United States by Frosch (1995), Busch (1995), and Auerbach (1993; Auerbach and Blatt, 1996).

Thus the notion of an intersubjectively acquired abstract reflexive implicit awareness of mental states, to be distinguished from intro-spection (Bolton and Hill, 1996), has always been at the core of many psychoanalytic formulations of self-development. The fruitful inte-gration of this classical idea with the relationship constructs of attachment theory serves to illustrate the potential of bringing psycho-analytic ideas to bear on attachment theory and, perhaps, vice versa.

(3) The Rediscovery of Psychoanalytic Ideas in Attachment Theory

It is inevitably a risky enterprise to draw parallels between concepts that emerge independently in different subject areas. The concept of "attachment" in sociology (Hirschi, 1969) refers to integration of the individual with a social structure and can only, with difficulty, be reduced to qualities of interpersonal relationships (Fonagy et al., 1997b). The same problem is encountered in linking concepts devel-oped in studies of attachment to psychoanalytic ideas based on clinical observations. The problem is compounded by the polymor-phous nature of most psychoanalytic ideas (Sandler, 1983) and their complex relations with the clinical evidence upon which they are based (Hamilton, 1996). There are other problems. Observations of attachment theorists are made based on experimental studies, at least in infancy, and relatively structured situations (interviews or questionnaires) in adulthood. It is not yet proven, and it is unlikely ever to be, that the parameters determining human behavior during free association in the consulting room are the same as those that pertain under conditions of controlled experimentation (Fonagy, 1982). The analogy between laboratory and clinically observed behavioral phenomena can therefore only be made at the level of mental processes: laboratory studies may help us identify the psychological mechanisms generating phenomena that become observable under clinical conditions. This principle applies to links between attachment and psychoanalytic theory. Are there any observations from the consulting room that may be helpfully elaborated in terms of constructs developed by attachment researchers? Conversely, are there observations made by attachment theorists that can be given and usefully expanded on the basis of psychoanalytic ideas generated in the clinical setting? Let us explore two possible instances of correspondence.

(1) *The concept of attachment:* Not surprisingly, attachment behaviors have been described by psychoanalysts using alternative terms that depict comparable phenomena. Perhaps the best example is Erikson's (1950) discussion of "basic trust." Based in drive theory, Erikson described the "incorporative" approach to life, which led the individual to establish patterns centered on the social modality of taking and holding onto objects physical and psychic. Erikson (1950) defined basic trust as the capacity "to receive and accept what is given" (p. 58). Careful reading of Erikson (1959) allows us to restate the classification of attachment security in Eriksonian terms. He ponders on the determinants of basic trust and discusses its dependence on the reception and acceptance of comforting from the primary caretaker. Mistrust (insecure attachment) may be caused by the inability to accept comfort and reassurance (resistance) or the withdrawing and in the extreme "closing up, refusing food and comfort and becoming oblivious to companionship" (p. 56) (avoidance). There are several further indications that "basic trust" is basically attachment. (i) Basic trust is derived from infantile experience, not mediated by oral gratification or demonstrations of love— rather by the quality of maternal relationships (Erikson, 1959, p. 63).

(ii) The failure of basic trust is the antecedent of whatever is the opposite of the "healthy personality" (Erikson, 1964). (iii) The notion of coherence of mental representation is the key to the way that basic trust may be transmitted across generations ("the experience of the caretaking person as a coherent human being") (Erikson, 1964, p. 117). (iv) Maternal sensitivity was seen as a key determinant of basic trust (Erikson, 1950). (v) Interactional synchrony (Isabella and Belsky, 1991) is similar to the Eriksonian description of "reciprocity or mutual regula-tion" (p. 58), while nonintrusive parenting (Malatesta et al., 1986) was described by Erikson in terms of the degree of control that the mother exerted.

There is a clear overlap between Erikson's thinking and Bowlby's observation. But Erikson is by no means the only psychoanalyst to arrive at the attachment construct. Anna Freud, a sworn enemy of attachment theory, clearly described attachment behaviors in her accounts of the impact of wartime separations on children (Freud, 1941–1945; Freud and Burlingham, 1944). More recently, Sandler's description of an inborn wish to maintain safety (Sandler, 1960, 1985) is analo-gous to Bowlby's emphasis on the innate propensity for attachment; the background of safety appears to be a phenomenological counterpart of the secure base concept. The abused child seeks contact with the abusing caretaker because, paradoxically, the predictable, familiar, but adverse experience has the potential to generate a greater sense of safety than an unfamiliar, nonabusive one.

A less obvious and potentially quite contentious analogy could be proposed between Klein's (1935) concept of the paranoid-schizoid position and insecurity of attachment. In the paranoid-schizoid position the relationship to the care-giver is represented as fragmented, split into persecutory and idealized relationships, and similarly the ego (the self) is assumed to be split. Only in the depressive position is the child thought to develop an integrated image of both loved and hated aspects of the parent and correspondingly do we see an integration of the self. There are facets of the description of insecure adult attachment (Main and Goldwyn, in press) that bring this category close to Klein's description of the paranoid-schizoid position. These might include: (i) The splitting of semantic and episodic memory, particularly in the dismissing category, is characterized by idealization and/or denigration of attachment figures. (ii) Lack of coherence or inconsistencies in relationship descriptions may be indicative of the lability of mental representation, which marks the paranoid-schizoid position (Klein, 1935). (iii) The balance of love and hate and the recognition and acceptance of imperfection in the caregiver is indicative of secure attachment and describes the state of mind characteristic of whole object perception in the depressive position (Klein, 1935). (iv) Secure attachment is marked by the individual's recall and recognition in bringing about interpersonal conflict and the generally enhanced capacity to monitor thoughts and feelings as these emerge in the narrative. Analogously in Klein's view, the onset of the depressive position is the child's discovery of his capacity to love and hate the parent, which opens the child to experiences of guilt (Klein, 1929). (v) The speech and discourse of secure individuals reflects superior symbolic capacity, and this may be linked to the association of symbolization to depressive reparation (Segal, 1957). (vi) Modern Kleinian writers see the critical aspect of the depressive position as the child's achievement of mental separateness and, linked to this the perception of the object as independent (Quinodox, 1991; Steiner, 1992). The same observation concerning the child's perception of the caregiver's independent functioning is made by Bowlby (1973).

What is suggested by the preceding list is not any kind of isomorphism between the concept of insecure attachment and the concept of a paranoid-schizoid state, but that the thinking of insecure adults may more frequently show features that have been described by Kleinian clinicians as paranoid-schizoid. Important implications may follow. For example, if it is accepted that paranoid-schizoid thinking is more prominent in insecure adults, this might imply that insecurity, rather than security, is the basic attachment position. The Kleinian perspective highlights an approach to attachment security as "a mode of mental functioning" with perhaps sometimes rapid cycling between secure and insecure modes (Bion, 1962b).

(2) *Attachment classification:* Psychoanalytic clinicians have described patterns of behavior and interpersonal relationship representations that correspond closely to classifications of adult attachment. Once again, such potential correspondences are important because of the alternative perspective psychoanalytic models cast on the mechanisms that could be mediating these individual differences.

Rosenfeld (1964, 1971a, b) distinguished between "thin skinned" and "thick skinned" narcissistic patterns. The clinical detail of his description resembles the preoccupied versus dismissing adult attachment categories. Using Rosenfeld's formulation we could see dismissing patterns of attachment as characterized by the tendency to deposit perceived inadequacies into others who are then experienced as under the control of the self given the assistance of projective identification. Preoccupied attachment could be identified psychoanalytically as associated with a sense of dependency that causes the individual to feel intolerable vulnerability to the other warded off through continuous angry attacks on those whose very dependability appears to mock the individual's feelings of helplessness. Those familiar with attachment classification will note that these descriptions cover only the angry resentful and the denigrating subcategories of the preoccupied and dismissing classifications, respectively.

Balint (1959) offered an alternative model for understanding the avoidant dismissing versus the resistant preoccupied patterns in his description of the "ocnophilic" and "philobatic" attitudes. In this formulation, the dismissing philobat is seen as the person who dislikes attachments but loves the spaces between them and who prefers to invest in his own ego skills at the expense of investing in his object. The preoccupied ocnophile defends against anxiety by enhancing his dependency on the newly emerging objects leading to an intensification of ambivalence. The dismissing attachment category may be similarly illuminated by Modell's (1975, 1984) formulation of narcissistic personality disorder.

Psychoanalytic ideas may also help elaborate upon our understanding of the disorganized attachment pattern of infancy (Main and Solomon, 1990). These children had been noted to manifest extraordinary controlling behavior in relation to their caregivers at preschool age (Cassidy, Marvin, and The MacArthur Working Group on Attachment, 1989) and in the early school years (Main and Cassidy, 1988). Children who were disorganized in their attachment in infancy, in separation–reunion situations, appear to take control of the relationship with their object, sometimes treating the parent in an apparently condescending or humiliating manner. Disorganized attachment has been shown to be associated with unresolved trauma in the parents (Main and Hesse, 1990), a history of maltreatment in the child (Carlsson et al., 1989), maternal depression (Radke-Yarrow et al., 1985), and parental substance abuse (Rodning, Beckwith, and Howard, 1991). We would argue that children exposed to such deprivation are repeatedly confronted with intolerable levels of confusing and hostile caregiving and commonly internalize images of the caregiver which they are incapable of integrating. The self-structure is thus formed incorporating fragmented and flawed images of the other, which the child is forced to externalize in order to retain an experience of coherence. The process of projective identification describes the behavior of such children well as they attempt to experience themselves as coherent selves and force unassimilable, "alien" parts of themselves into the other. They confirm this illusion by more or less subtle manipulative control over the other's behavior, ensuring that the perception of these alien aspects of the self as being external can be maintained (Fonagy and Target, 1997).

Some Specific Areas Where Attachment Theory Could Benefit From Psychoanalytic Insights

It would be foolhardy to maintain that psychoanalytic critiques of attachment theory are altogether misguided. In important respects psychoanalytic formulations are significantly in advance of the understanding that attachment theory is able to provide. A more complete integration of psychoanalytic and attachment theory would demand that attachment researchers address these areas of discrepancy and elaborate on their formulations in the direction of making them more compatible with a psychoanalytic framework.

What are the shortcomings of current attachment theory from a psychoanalytic standpoint? First, attachment theory should pay more attention to systematic distortions in the child's perceptions of the external world. The relationship of actual experience and its representation is greatly complicated by the fact that comparable caregiver behavior may be experienced and encoded differently by different infants (Eagle, 1997). While contextual factors, for example, small differences between the caregiver's behavior toward two siblings (nonshared environment), may account for some of these effects, distortions in the child's perception because of internal states of fantasies, affects, and conflicts are also likely to play a part.

Second, internal working models are probably often in conflict, vying for dominance for organization of a particular relationship. They are also likely to exist in a hierarchy, some with greater access to consciousness than others. Even if these models are solely encoded as procedures, that is, are implicit rather than explicit, it is probable that they will vary in terms of their developmental appropriateness, some appearing to be age-appropriate while others represent immature, regressive ways of relating. Interestingly, the developmental dimension of attachment theory is limited. While it is self-evident that adult manifestations of, say avoidance, must be different from the manifestation of this class of attachments in adolescence, work thus far has focused on the identification of continuities between these manifestations rather than expectable developmental changes, which are likely to accompany the maturational differentiation of the child's representational system. Since Freud (1900), psychoanalytic developmentalists have always been concerned by how self, object, and object relationship representations evolve with development (Jacobson, 1964; Freud, 1965; Mahler, Pine, and Bergman, 1975). Internal working models are likely to become marked by the mode and level of functioning prevalent at the time of their construction. The amount of interpersonal awareness or self–other differentiation shown by an individual may be a factor of attachment class, but it also may indicate the developmental level of the representational model.

A third and related developmental issue concerns discontinuities of attachment classification. Attachment theorists prefer to conceive of such discontinuities in terms of environmental changes. They rarely ask the question why environmental changes do not invariably impact on the attachment system. Psychoanalysts have also shown considerable sophistication in the way that the same developmental influence, for example, sensitivity, may have quite a different impact on relationship representations at different developmental stages.

Fourth, psychoanalytic objections to attachment theory often focus on the allegedly simplistic categorical system attachment theory offers. This is a misunderstanding and reflects the conflation in the mind of critics of the operationalization of a theory with the theory itself. The criticism, however, is warranted to the extent that attachment researchers often appear to reify attachment categories and consider them as theoretical entities rather than observed clusters of behavior. A problem arises if researchers cease to concern themselves with the mechanisms or psychic processes that may underlie such behavioral clusters. Beginning to think about these groupings more in psychoanalytic terms, whether as habitual modes of defense or as manifestations of a representational system overinfluenced by paranoid-schizoid modes of functioning, might reduce the danger of the reification of attachment categories. The psychoanalytic perspective might encourage us to think less categorically and more dimensionally about attachment security. The potential for both security and insecurity is likely to be present in all of us.

Fifth, psychoanalytic concern with the development of the child's awareness of the integrity of his object could direct the attachment researcher's attention to the biological role of attachment. Bowlby's classical assumption, that attachment behavior has a selective advantage as it promotes the survival of the species, is inconsistent with the advances of sociobiology and behavior genetics. "The survival of the species" is not what drives evolution. It is the survival of the genetic code carried by a particular individual that is at an evolutionary premium. So what is the selection advantage of a social protective mechanism based on the expression of distress in the infant? The answer is not obvious, since we now recognize that the expression of distress carries a high risk for the infant. The work of Bruce Perry (1997) illustrates how neglect, in arousing a chronic fright–flight reaction, has the potential to cause significant neurodevelopmental anomalies (because of the presence of excessive cortisol in the brain). The fright–flight reaction in such infants is thus evolutionarily a high-risk strategy, the purpose of which is unclear since the infant is unable to respond to threat by either of these methods. Surely, a simpler, less distressing, and therefore less risky method of signaling danger could have evolved. The caregiver's attachment system could be activated by an innate releasing mechanism that was neutral to the infant's well-being.

Taking a psychoanalytic perspective might illuminate this evolutionary puzzle. The infant's distress not only brings the caregiver physically close to the child but also creates comparable distress in the object. Thus, an ideal situation is created for the infant to experience containment (Bion, 1962a) and accurate mirroring (Winnicott, 1967), in other words, a context within which internalization processes essential to self-development can take place. The evolutionary function of the attachment system thus may not be self-evident as Bowlby thought, the eliciting of a protective response from a human adult. Instead, the survival risks to the organism entailed in the processes of attachment are justified by the benefit that the experience of psychic containment brings in terms of the development of a coherent and symbolizing self. There is evidence that secure attachment in infancy and the experience of sensitive caregiving upon which this is likely to be based predicts superior capacity to understand the nature of mental states (Fonagy et al., 1997a, submitted). It is therefore at least plausible to argue that at least one biological function of the processes of attachment is the creation of a particular intersubjective environment. Here, the proximity of the caregiver, in the state of arousal concordant with that of the child, permits an internalization of that mental state that can become the root of a second-order representation of this state of distress and ultimately permit symbolic understanding of internal states by the human mind (Gergely and Watson, 1996).

Finally, complementary to the addition of a psychoanalytic perspective to developmental attachment theory, psychoanalytic ideas could greatly enrich attachment theory formulations of psychopathology. To take the example of borderline personality disorder, Kernberg's (1975, 1977) description of borderline personality organization could be seen in attachment theory terms as a lack of integration of internal working models or, rather, the predominance of internal working models where self and object representations rapidly oscillate. Attachment theory needs to learn more about the incomplete internal working models with which such individuals function. The relationship representation is not that with an actual other but, rather, a small fragment of that person experienced at a moment characterized by overwhelming and diffuse affect. Insecure attachment with accompanying inadequate affect regulation is bound to increase the likelihood of the creation of such partial internal working models. There is evidence from studies of borderline patients, using the adult attachment interview, of a characteristic dominance of confusing and confused internal representations of attachment (Patrick et al., 1994; Fonagy et al., 1996). Kernberg's clinical formulation implies the presence of easily activated, poorly structured, highly distorted partial and unstable internal working models in such individuals with characteristically loose assignments of objects and subjects. Rapid alteration between working models, as well as the absence of coherence within them, may be associated with an inhibition of a metacognitive or reflective capacity that normally serves the function of self-organization (Fonagy and Target, 1997). The abandonment of reflective function may be seen as constitutional or as an extreme defensive response of children confronted with traumatic situations where they might find overwhelming the contemplation of mental states in their caregiver or themselves. They thus voluntarily abandon this crucial psychological capacity, with sometimes disastrous consequences.

Conclusion

Attachment theory and psychoanalytic theory have common roots but have evolved in epistemologically distinct ways. Attachment theory, far closer to empirical psychology with its positivist heritage, has been in some ways method-bound over the past 15 years. Its scope was determined less by what fell within the domain defined by relationship phenomena involving a caretaking-dependent dyad and more by the range of groups and behaviors to which the preferred mode of observation, the strange situation, the adult attachment interview, and so forth, could be productively applied. This sheltered the theory from a range of ideas that clinical psychoanalysts evolved, particularly in the context of analytic work with increasingly severely disturbed chronic personality-disordered individuals.

Psychoanalytic ideas have rarely taken into consideration relevant observations from the field of attachment, and conversely, a paradigm-bound attachment theory has felt it had little to benefit from the clinical discoveries of psychoanalysts. Yet both bodies of knowledge are progressing toward the same end-point, which is perhaps still some way off: a developmental understanding of personality and psychological disorder. This paper attempted to illustrate that distinctions made by attachment theorists are frequently closely linked to distinctions generally accepted within particular psychoanalytic traditions. Attachment theory may share more with some psychoanalytic traditions than others, but this does not mean that even "distant cousins" of attachment theory (e.g., modern Kleinian theory) do not cover similar ground, albeit from a radically different perspective. Taking psychoanalytic theory as a whole, many important discoveries of attachment theory could be seen to have been observed on the couch as well as in the laboratory.

There are some areas familiar to psychoanalytic clinicians where attachment theory has not yet ventured. Bringing the two approaches into closer contact, beyond creating lively debate, has the potential to enrich both traditions greatly. It may highlight where attachment theory methodology may be applied for the exploration of psychoanalytic work and ideas. For example, attachment status may be used as a measure of outcome for psychoanalytic treatment. The focus of attachment research may additionally be broadened to incorporate areas beyond its traditional domain of social development in the context of the dyad.

REFERENCES

Auerbach, J. S. (1993), The origins of narcissism and narcissistic personality disorder: A theoretical and empirical reformulation. In: *Psychoanalytic Perspectives on Psychopathology*, J. M. Masling & R. F. Bornstein. Washington, DC: American Psychological Association, pp. 43–110.

———— & Blatt, S. J. (1996), Self-representation in severe psychopathology: The role of reflexive self-awareness. *Psychoanal. Psychol.*, 13:297–341.

Balint, M. (1952), On love and hate. *Internat. J. Psycho-Anal.*, 33:355–362.

———— (1959), *Thrills and Regressions*. London: Hogarth Press.

Bion, W. R. (1959), Attacks on linking. *Internat. J. Psycho-Anal.*, 40:308–315.

———— (1962a), *Learning from Experience*. London: Heinemann.

———— (1962b), A theory of thinking. *Internat. J. Psycho-Anal.*, 43:306–310.

———— (1967), *Second Thoughts*. London: Heinemann.

Bolton, D., & Hill, J. (1996), *Mind, Meaning and Mental Disorder*. Oxford: Oxford University Press.

Bowlby, J. (1946), *Forty-four Juvenile Thieves: Their Character and Homelife*. London: Balliere, Tyndall & Cox.

———— (1958), The nature of the child's tie to his mother. *Internat. J. Psycho-Anal.*, 39:350–373.

———— (1960), Grief and mourning in infancy and early childhood. *The Psychoanalytic Study of the Child*, 15:3–39. New York: International Universities Press.

———— (1969), *Attachment and Loss, Vol. 1: Attachment*. London: Hogarth Press.

———— (1973), *Attachment and Loss, Vol. 2: Separation: Anxiety and Anger*. London: Hogarth Press.

———— (1977), The making and breaking of affectional bonds II: Some principles of psychotherapy. *Brit. J. Psychiat.*, 130:421–431.

———— (1980a), *Attachment and Loss, Vol. 3: Loss: Sadness and Depression*. London: Hogarth Press.

———— (1980b), Epilogue. In: *The Place of Attachment in Human Behaviour*, ed. C. M. Parks & J. Stevenson-Hinde. New York: Basic Books, pp. 301–312.

Bretherton, I. (1987), New perspectives on attachment relationships: Security, communication and internal working models. In: *Handbook of Infant Development*, ed. J. D. Osofsky. New York: Wiley, pp. 1061–1100.

———— (1995), Internal working models: Cognitive and affective aspects of attachment representations. In: *4th Rochester Symposium on Developmental Psychopathology on "Emotion, Cognition, and Representation,"* ed. D. Cicchetti & S. Toth. Hillsdale, NJ: Lawrence Erlbaum.

———— Bates, E., Benigni, L., Camaioni, L. & Volterra, V. (1979), Relationships between cognition, communication, and quality of attachment. In: *The Emergence of Symbols*, ed. E. Bates, L. Benigni, I. Bretherton, L. Camaioni & V. Volterra. New York: Academic Press.

Bucci, W. (1997), *Psychoanalysis and Cognitive Science: A Multiple Code Theory*. New York: Guilford Press.

Busch, F. (1995), Do actions speak louder than words? A query into an enigma in analytic theory and technique. *J. Amer. Psychoanal. Assn.* 43:61–82.

Carlsson, E. & Sroufe, L. A. (1995), Contribution of attachment theory to developmental psychopathology. In: *Developmental Psychopathology. Vol. 1: Theory and Methods*, ed. D. Cicchetti & D. J. Cohen. New York: Wiley, pp. 581–617.

Carlsson, V., Cicchetti, D., Barnett, D. & Braunwald, K. (1989), Disorganised/disoriented attachment relationships in maltreated infants. *Devel. Psychol.*, 25:525–531.

Cassidy, J. (1994), Emotion regulation: Influences of attachment research. *Monographs of the Society for Research in Child Development* (Serial No 240), 59:228–283.

———— Marvin, R. S. & MacArthur Working Group (1989), *Attachment Organization in Three and Four Year Olds: Coding Guidelines*. University of Illinois. Unpublished.

Crittenden, P. M. (1990), Internal representational models of attachment relationships. *J. Inf. Mental Hlth.,* 11:259–277.

De Wolff, M. S. & van IJzendoorn, M. H. (1997), Sensitivity and attachment: A meta-analysis on parental antecedents of infant attachment. *Child Devel.,* 68:571–591.

Dunn, J. (1996), The Emanuel Miller Memorial Lecture 1995. Children's relationships: Bridging the divide between cognitive and social development. *J. Child Psychol. & Psychiat.,* 37:507–518.

Eagle, M. (1995), The developmental perspectives of attachment and psychoanalytic theory. In: *Attachment Theory: Social, Developmental and Clinical Perspectives,* ed. S. Goldberg, R. Muir & J. Kerr. Hillsdale, NJ: The Analytic Press, pp. 123–150.

——— (1997), Attachment and psychoanalysis. *Brit. J. Med. Psychol.,* 70:217–229.

Engel, G. L. (1971), Attachment behaviour, object relations and the dynamic point of view. A critical review of Bowlby's Attachment and Loss. *Internat. J. Psycho-Anal.,* 52:183–196.

Erikson, E. H. (1950), *Childhood and Society.* New York: Norton.

——— (1959), *Identity and the Life Cycle.* New York: International Universities Press.

——— (1964), *Insight and Responsibility.* New York: Norton.

——— (1968), *Identity, Youth and Crisis.* New York: Norton.

Fairbairn, W. R. D. (1952), *An Object-Relations Theory of the Personality.* New York: Basic Books.

Ferenczi, S. (1933), A confusion of tongues between adults and the child. In: *Final Contributions to the Problems and Methods of Psychoanalysis,* ed. M. Balint. London: Hogarth Press, 1955, pp. 156–167.

Fonagy, P. (1982), Psychoanalysis and empirical science. *Internat. Rev. Psycho-Anal.,* 9:125–145.

——— Leigh, T., Steele, M., Steele, H., Kennedy, R., Mattoon, G., Target, M. & Gerber, A. (1996), The relation of attachment status, psychiatric classification, and response to psychotherapy. *J. Consult. & Clin. Psychol.,* 64:22–31.

——— Redfern, S. & Charman, T. (1997a), The relationship between belief-desire reasoning and a projective measure of attachment security (SAT). *Brit. J. Devel. Psychol.,* 15:51–61.

——— Steele, H., Moran, G., Steele, M. & Higgitt, A. (1991), The capacity for understanding mental states: The reflective self in parent and child and its significance for security of attachment. *Inf. Mental Hlth. J.,* 13:200–217.

——— ——— Steele, M. & Holder, J. (submitted), Quality of attachment to mother at one year predicts belief-desire reasoning at 5 years. *Child Devel.*

——— ——— ——— ——— ——— ——— ——— Leigh, T., Kennedy, R., Mattoon, G. & Target, M. (1995a), Attachment, the reflective self, and borderline states: The predictive specificity of the Adult Attachment Interview and pathological emotional development. In: *Attachment Theory: Social, Developmental and Clinical Perspectives,* ed. S. Goldberg, R. Muir & J. Kerr. Hillsdale, NJ: The Analytic Press, pp. 233–278.

——— ——— ——— ——— ——— ——— ——— (1995b), The predictive validity of Mary Main's Adult Attachment Interview: A psychoanalytic and developmental perspective on the transgenerational transmission of attachment and borderline states. In: *Attachment Theory; Social, Developmental and Clinical Perspectives,* ed. S. Goldberg, R. Muir, & J. Kerr. Hillsdale, NJ: The Analytic Press, pp. 233–278.

———— & Target, M. (1997), Attachment and reflective function: Their role in self-organization. *Devel. & Psychopathol.,* 9:679–700.

———— ———— Steele, M., Steele, H., Leigh, T., Levinson, A. & Kennedy, R. (1997b), Crime and attachment: Morality, disruptive behaviour, borderline personality disorder, crime and their relationship to security of attachment. In: *Attachment and Psychopathology,* ed. L. Atkinson & K. J. Zucker. New York: Guilford Press, pp. 223–274.

Fraiberg, S. (1982), Pathological defenses in infancy. *Psychoanal. Quart.,* 51:612–635.

Freud, A. (1936), *The Ego and the Mechanisms of Defence.* New York: International Universities Press, 1946.

———— (1941–1945), Reports on the Hampstead Nurseries, *The Writings of Anna Freud.* New York: International Universities Press, 1974.

———— (1954), The widening scope of indications for psychoanalysis: discussion. *J. Amer. Psychoanal. Assn.,* 2:607–620.

———— (1955), The concept of the rejecting mother, *The Writings of Anna Freud.* New York: International Universities Press, pp. 586–602, 1968.

———— (1960), Discussion of Dr. Bowlby's paper (Grief and mourning in infancy and early childhood), *The Writings of Anna Freud.* New York: International Universities Press, pp. 167–186, 1969.

———— (1965), *Normality and Pathology in Childhood.* Harmondsworth: Penguin Books.

———— & Burlingham, D. (1944), *Infants Without Families.* New York: International Universitics Press.

Freud, S. (1900), The interpretation of dreams. *Standard Edition,* 4,5:1–625. London: Hogarth Press, 1953.

———— (1911), Formulations on the two principles of mental functioning. *Standard Edition,* 12:218–226. London: Hogarth Press, 1958.

———— (1917), Introductory lectures on psycho-analysis: Part III. General theory of the neuroses. *Standard Edition,* 17:7–122. London: Hogarth Press, 1955.

———— (1923), The ego and the id. *Standard Edition,* 19:12–66. London: Hogarth Press, 1961.

———— (1926), Inhibitions, symptoms and anxiety. *Standard Edition,* 20:87–175. London: Hogarth Press, 1959.

———— (1931), Female sexuality. *Standard Edition,* 21:225–243. London: Hogarth Press, 1961.

———— (1939), Moses and monotheism. *Standard Edition* 23:3–137. London: Hogarth Press, 1964.

Frosch, A. (1995), The preconceptual organization of emotion. *J. Amer. Psychoanal. Assn.,* 43:423–447.

Gergely, G. (1992), Developmental reconstructions: Infancy from the point of view of psychoanalysis and developmental psychology. *Psychoanal. & Contemp. Thought,* 14:3–55.

———— (submitted), Reapproaching Mahler: New perspectives on normal autism, normal symbiosis, splitting and libidinal object constancy from cognitive developmental theory. *J. Amer. Psychoanal. Assn.*

———— & Watson, J. (1996), The social biofeedback model of parental affect-mirroring. *Internat. J. Psycho-Anal.,* 77:1181–1212.

Green, A. (1975), The analyst, symbolisation and absence in the analytic setting: On changes in analytic practice and analytic experience. *Internat. J. Psycho-Anal.*, 56:1–22.

Greenacre, P. (1952), Pregenital patterning. *Internat. J. Psycho-Anal.*, 33:410–415.

Grosskruth, P. (1986), *Melanie Klein: Her World and Her Work.* New York: Knopf.

Guntrip, H. (1961), *Personality Structure and Human Interaction.* New York: International Universities Press.

Hamilton, V. (1996), *The Analyst's Preconscious.* Hillsdale, NJ: The Analytic Press.

Hanly, C. (1978), A critical consideration of Bowlby's ethological theory of anxiety. *Psychoanal. Quart.*, 47:364–380.

Hirschi, T. (1969), *Causes of Delinquency.* Berkeley, CA: University of California Press.

Holmes, J. (1993), *John Bowlby and Attachment Theory.* London: Routledge.

———— (1997), Attachment, autonomy, intimacy: Some clinical implications of attachment theory. *Brit. J. Med. Psychol.*, 70:231–248.

Isabella, R. & Belsky, J. (1991a), Interactional synchrony and the origins of infant-mother attachment: A replication study. *Child Dev.*, 62:373–384.

Jacobson, E. (1954), The self and the object world: Vicissitudes of their infantile cathexes and their influence on ideational affective development. *The Psychoanalytic Study of the Child*, 9:75–127. International Universities Press.

———— (1964), *The Self and the Object World.* New York: International Universities Press.

Kernberg, O. F. (1975), *Borderline Conditions and Pathological Narcissism.* New York: Aronson.

———— (1976a), *Object Relations Theory and Clinical Psychoanalysis.* New York: Aronson.

———— (1976b), Technical considerations in the treatment of borderline personality organisation. *J. Amer. Psychoanal. Assn.*, 24:795–829.

———— (1977), The structural diagnosis of borderline personality organization. In: *Borderline Personality Disorders: The Concept, the Syndrome, the Patient*, ed. P. Hartocollis. New York: International Universities Press, pp. 87–121.

Klein, M. (1929), Infantile anxiety-situations reflected in a work of art and in the creative impulse. In: *Contributions to Psychoanalysis, 1921–1945*, ed. New York: McGraw-Hill, 1964, pp. 156–167.

———— (1935), A contribution to the psychogenesis of manic-depressive states. In: *The Writings of Melanie Klein*, ed. R. Money-Kyrie. London: Hogarth Press, 1975, pp. 236–289.

———— (1945), The Oedipus complex in the light of early anxieties. *The Writings of Melanie Klein*, ed. R. Money-Kyrie. London: Hogarth Press, 1975, pp. 370–419.

———— (1981), On Mahler's autistic and symbiotic phases: An exposition and evaluation. *Psychoanal. & Contemp. Thought*, 4:69–105.

Kohut, H. (1971), *The Analysis of the Self.* New York: International Universities Press.

———— (1977), *The Restoration of the Self.* New York: International Universities Press.

———— & Wolf, E. S. (1978), The disorders of the self and their treatment: An outline. *Internat. J. Psycho-Anal.*, 59:413–425.

Lichtenberg, J. (1989), *Psychoanalysis and Motivation.* Hillsdale, NJ: The Analytic Press.

———— (1995), Can empirical studies of development impact on psychoanalytic theory and technique? In: *Research in Psychoanalysis: Process, Development, Outcome*, ed. T. Shapiro & R. N. Emde. New York: International Universities Press, pp. 261–276.

Luquet, P. (1981), Le changement dans la mentalization. *Rev. Français de Psychoanal.*, 45:1023–1028.

———— (1987), Penser-Parler: Un apport psychanalytique à la théorie du langage. In: *La Parole Troublée*, ed. R. Christie, M. M. Christie-Luterbacher, & P. Luquet. Paris: Presses Universitaire de France, pp. 161–300.

———— (1988), Langage, pensée et structure psychique. *Rev. Français Psychoanal.*, 52:267–302.

Mahler, M. S., Pine, F. & Bergman, A. (1975), *The Psychological Birth of the Human Infant: Symbiosis and Individuation*. New York: Basic Books.

Main, M. (1991), Metacognitive knowledge, metacognitive monitoring, and singular (coherent) vs. multiple (incoherent) model of attachment: Findings and directions for future research. In: *Attachment Across the Life Cycle*, ed. C. M. Parkes, J. Stevenson-Hinde, & P. Marris. London: Tavistock/Routledge, pp. 127–159.

———— & Cassidy, J. (1988), Categories of response to reunion with the parent at age 6: Predictable from infant attachment classifications and stable over a 1-month period. *Devel. Psychol.*, 24:415–426.

———— & Goldwyn, R. (in press), Adult attachment classification system. In: *Behavior and the Development of Representational Models of Attachment: Five Methods of Assessment*, ed. M. Main. New York: Cambridge University Press.

———— & Goldwyn, R. (in preparation), Adult attachment rating and classification systems. In: *A Typology of Human Attachment Organization Assessed in Discourse, Drawings and Interviews* (working title), ed. M. Main. New York: Cambridge University Press.

———— & Hesse, E. (1990), Parents' unresolved traumatic experiences are related to infant disorganized attachment status: Is frightened and/or frightening parental behavior the linking mechanism? In: *Attachment in the Preschool Years: Theory, Research and Intervention*, ed. M. Greenberg, D. Cicchetti & E. M. Cummings. Chicago: University of Chicago Press, pp. 161–182.

———— Kaplan, N. & Cassidy, J. (1985), Security in infancy, childhood and adulthood: A move to the level of representation. In: *Growing Points of Attachment Theory and Research. Monographs of the Society for Research in Child Development, Vol. 50*, ed. I. Bretherton & E. Waters. Chicago: Chicago University Press, pp. 66–104.

———— & Solomon, J. (1990), Procedures for identifying infants as disorganized/disoriented during the Ainsworth Strange Situation. In: *Attachment During the Preschool Years: Theory, Research and Intervention*, ed. D. C. M. Greenberg & E. M. Cummings. Chicago: University of Chicago Press, pp. 121–160.

Malatesta, C. Z., Grigoryev, P., Lamb, C., Albin, M. & Culver, C. (1986), Emotional socialisation and expressive development in pre-term and full-term infants. *Child Devel.*, 57:316–330.

Marty, P. (1968), A major process of somatization: The progressive disorganization. *Internat. J. Psycho-Anal.*, 49:246–249.

———— (1990), *La Psychsomatique de l'Adulte*. Paris: Presses Universitaires de France.

———— (1991), *Mentalization et Psychsomatique*. Paris: Laboratoire Delagrange.

Masson, J. (1984), *The Assault on Truth: Freud's Suppression of the Seduction Theory.* New York: Farrar, Straus & Giroux.

McDougall, J. (1978), *Plea for a Measure of Abnormality.* New York: International Universities Press.

Meins, E. & Russell, J. (1997), Security and symbolic play: The relation between security of attachment and executive capacity. *Brit. J. Dev. Psychol.,* 15:63–76.

Modell, A. (1975), A narcissistic defense against affects and the illusion of self-sufficiency. *Internat. J. Psycho-Anal.,* 56:275–282.

——— (1984), *Psychoanalysis in a New Context.* New York: International Universities Press.

Morgan, A. C. (1998), Moving along to things left undone. *J. Inf. Mental Hlth.,* 19:324–332.

Morton, J. & Frith, U. (1995), Causal modeling: A structural approach to developmental psychology. In: *Developmental Psychopathology. Vol. 1: Theory and Methods,* ed. D. Cicchetti & D. J. Cohen. New York: John Wiley, pp. 357–390.

Moss, E., Parent, S. & Gosselin, C. (1995), Attachment and theory of mind: Cognitive and metacognitive correlates of attachment during the preschool period. Paper presented at the the biennial meeting of the Society for Research in Child Development, Indianapolis, IN, March–April.

Patrick, M., Hobson, R. P., Castle, D., Howard, R. & Maughan, B. (1994), Personality disorder and the mental representation of early social experience. *Dev. Psychopathol.,* 6:375–388.

Perry, B. (1997), Incubated in terror: Neurodevelopmental factors in the "cycle of violence." In: *Children in a Violent Society,* ed. J. Osofsky. New York: Guilford Press, pp. 124–149.

Quinodox, J. M. (1991), Accepting fusion to get over it. *Rev. Français Psychoanal.,* 55:1697–1700.

Radke-Yarrow, M., Cummings, E. M., Kuczynski, L. & Chapman, M. (1985), Patterns of attachment in two- and three-year-olds in normal families and families with parental depression. *Child Devel.,* 56:884–893.

Rochlin, G. (1971), Review of Bowlby, J., Attachment and loss: Attachment. *Psychoanal. Quart.,* 50:504–506.

Rodning, C., Beckwith, L. & Howard, J. (1991), Quality of attachment and home environment in children prenatally exposed to PCP and cocaine. *Devel. & Psychopathol.,* 3:351–366.

Roiphe, H. (1976), Review of J. Bowlby, Attachment and loss. II: Separation, anxiety and anger. *Psychoanal. Quart.,* 65:307–309.

Rosenfeld, H. (1964), On the psychopathology of narcissism: A clinical approach. *Internat. J. Psycho-Anal.,* 45:332–337.

——— (1971a), A clinical approach to the psychoanalytic theory of the life and death instincts: An investigation into to the aggressive aspects of narcissism. *Internat. J. Psycho-Anal.,* 52:169–178.

——— (1971b), Contribution to the psychopathology of psychotic states: The importance of projective identification in the ego structure and object relations of the psychotic patient. In: *Melanie Klein Today,* ed. E. B. Spillius. London: Routledge, 1988, pp. 117–137.

Sander, L. (in press), Interventions that effect therapeutic change. *J. Inf. Mental Hlth.*

Sandler, J. (1960), The background of safety. *From Safety to Superego: Selected Papers of Joseph Sandler*. London: Karnac, 1987, pp. 1–8.

——— (1976), Actualisation and object relationships. *J. Phila. Assn. Psychoanal.*, 3:59–70.

——— (1983), Reflections on some relations between psychoanalytic concepts and psychoanalytic practice. *Internat. J. Psycho-Anal.*, 64:35–45.

——— (1985), Towards a reconsideration of the psychoanalytic theory of motivation. *Bull. Anna Freud Centre*, 8:223–243.

——— (1987a), The concept of projective identification. In: *Projection, Identification, Projection Identification*, ed. J. Sandler. Madison, CT: International Universities Press, pp. 13–26.

——— (1987b), *Projection, Identification, Projective Identification*. London: Karnac Books.

——— & Rosenblatt, B. (1962), The representational world. In: *From Safety to Superego. Selected Papers of Joseph Sandler*, ed. J. Sandler. London: Karnac Books, 1987, pp. 58–72.

Schacter, D. L. (1992), Understanding implicit memory: A cognitive neuroscience approach. *Amer. Psychol.*, 47:559–569.

Schafer, R. (1983), *The Analytic Attitude*. New York: Basic Books.

Schur, M. (1960), Discussion of Dr. John Bowlby's paper. *The Psychoanalytic Study of the Child*, 15:63–84. New York: International Universities Press.

Segal, H. (1957), Notes on symbol formation. *Internat. J. Psycho-Anal.*, 38:391–397.

Shane, M., Shane, E. & Gales, M. (1997), *Intimate Attachments: Toward a New Self Psychology*. New York: Guilford Press.

Spitz, R. (1945), Hospitalism: An inquiry into the genesis of psychiatric conditions in early childhood. *The Psychoanalytic Study of the Child*, 1:53–73. New York: International Universities Press.

——— (1965), *The First Year of Life*. New York: International Universities Press.

——— (1959), *A Genetic Field Theory of Ego Formation: Its Implications for Pathology*. New York: International Universities Press.

——— (1960), Discussion of Dr. John Bowlby's paper. *The Psychoanalytic Study of the Child*, *15*, 85–94. New York: International Universities Press.

Sroufe, L. A. (1990), An organizational perspective on the self. In: *The Self in Transition: Infancy to Childhood*, ed. D. Cicchetti & M. Beeghly. Chicago: University of Chicago Press, pp. 281–307.

——— (1996), *Emotional Development: The Organization of Emotional Life in the Early Years*. New York: Cambridge University Press.

Steiner, J. (1992), The equilibrium between the paranoid-schizoid and the depressive positions. In: *Clinical Lectures on Klein and Bion*, ed. R. Anderson. London: Routledge, pp. 46–58.

Stern, D. J. (1994), One way to build a clinically relevant baby. *Inf. Mental Hlth. J.*, 15:36–54.

Stern, D. N. (1985), *The Interpersonal World of the Infant: A View from Psychoanalysis and Developmental Psychology*. New York: Basic Books.

——— (1998), The process of therapeutic change involving implicit knowledge: Some implications of developmental observations for adult psychotherapy. *Inf. Mental Hlth. J.*, 19:300–308.

Tronick, E. Z. (1998), Dyadically expanded states of consciousness and the process of therapeutic change. *Inf. Mental Hlth. J.,* 19:290–299.

Winnicott, D. W. (1953), Transitional objects and transitional phenomena. *Internat. J. Psycho-Anal.,* 34:1–9.

———— (1956), Mirror role of mother and family in child development. In: *Playing and Reality,* by D. W. Winnicott. London: Tavistock, pp. 111–118.

———— (1962), Ego integration in child development. In: .. *The Maturational Processes and the Facilitating Environment,* by D. W. Winnicott. London: Hogarth Press, 1965, pp. 56–63.

———— (1965), *The Maturational Process and the Facilitating Environment.* London: Hogarth Press.

———— (1967), Mirror-role of the mother and family in child development. In: *The Predicament of the Family: A Psycho-Analytical Symposium,* ed. P. Lomas. London: Hogarth Press, pp. 26–33.

Yorke, C. (1971), Some suggestions for a critique of Kleinian psychology. *The Psychoanalytic Study of the Child,* 26:129–155. New York: International Universities Press.

Sub-Department of Clinical Health Psychology
University College London
Gower Street, London WC1E 6BT
E-mail: p.fonagy@ucl.ac.uk

Second-Generation Effects of Unresolved Trauma in Nonmaltreating Parents: Dissociated, Frightened, and Threatening Parental Behavior

ERIK HESSE, Ph.D.
MARY MAIN, Ph.D.

. . . it is certain that the problem of fear is the meeting point of many important questions, an enigma whose complete solution would cast a flood of light upon psychic life.

—S. Freud, 1920, p. 340

ATTACHMENT THEORY ORIGINATED within the domain of psycho-analysis, and like much of psychoanalytic theory examines the influence of early development upon both healthy and pathological forms of psychological functioning (Bowlby, 1969). Both attachment theory and its accompanying research paradigms differ from tradi-tional psychoanalytic perspectives, however, in (a) focusing on the evolutionary origins or the adaptive (biological) function of the child's

Dr. Hesse is director of the Social Development Project in the Department of Psychology at the University of California at Berkeley, and is an Adjunct Scientist at the Center for Child and Family Studies, Leiden University.

Dr. Main is a professor in developmental and biological psychology in the Department of Psychology at the University of California at Berkeley.

This paper is dedicated to the memory of our friend Joseph Sandler, whose "safety principle" is closely related to the central themes within this work. We thank Sydney Blatt, Diana Diamond, Sarah Hesse, Joseph Lichtenberg, and Marinus van IJzendoorn for remarks and suggestions which led to substantial improvements in this presentation. We are grateful to the American Psychoanalytic Foundation, the Harris Foundation of Chicago, and the Kohler-Stiftung foundation of Munich for their financial assistance in support of this project.

tie to its mother and relatedly, (b) encouraging a simultaneously ethological and experimental approach to research. Early research in attachment had perhaps rightly been criticized for placing too great an emphasis on the observation of behavior at the expense of an examination of internal processes. In recent years, however, significant progress has been made within the field of attachment, and ways of systematically approaching the study of representational processes in children and in adults have been developed (Main, Kaplan and Cassidy, 1985).

As a result, research in attachment has gained the increasing attention of adult and child clinicians. This is no doubt due in part to the creation of language-based methodologies—for example, the Adult Attachment Interview, with its emphasis upon individual differences in language usage during the discussion of past experiences—which has advanced the potential for designing and testing clinical hypotheses in adults, and more recently in latency-aged children as well[1] (AAI, George, Kaplan, and Main, 1984, 1985, 1996; Main and Goldwyn, 1984–1998; see Hesse, 1999a, for overview). Concurrently, fine-grained research into the behavior of parents and infants has continued to be conducted against the backdrop of the Ainsworth strange situation procedure (Ainsworth et al., 1978) and its middle-childhood equivalents (Main and Cassidy, 1988), in addition to other laboratory and home observation(s) of parent-offspring interactions. By combining these methodologies, researchers are beginning to investigate relations between representational processes in caregivers, and behavioral and (later) representational processes in their offspring. It

---

[1] As Hesse's (1999a) overview indicates, three studies employing the AAI with children have been successfully carried out. Maureen Gaffney at Trinity College has recently reported that interviews conducted with 11 year old children in Dublin (N = 22) have a 77% secure vs. insecure match to those of their mothers, a finding virtually identical to the average match previously reported in a meta-analysis of mother-infant samples (van IJzendoorn, 1995). Ammaniti and his colleagues at the University of Rome have found secure vs. insecure attachment status stable from 10 to 14 years of age, while in a blind study Judith Trowell and her colleagues at the Tavistock Clinic in London have found the AAI categories sharply discriminated 42 sexually abused children (6-14 years) from their matched (20 community and 20 community mental health controls. All three research groups have used the Main and Goldwyn (1984–1998) system of interview analysis. Trowell (personal communication, 1999) finds that the full interview works well with children 9 years of age and older, but understanding queries regarding past experiences seemed difficult for those 6 to 8 year olds independently exhibiting deficits in language comprehension.

is therefore gradually becoming possible to systematize the precursors to a variety of clinical outcomes.

Using traditional attachment theory as well as some of its more recent extensions, this presentation focuses upon the confusing, disorganizing and disorienting effects which repeated experiences involving fear of the parent are likely to engender among attached infants. In some cases, of course, an infant will be fearful of the parent as a result of physical abuse. Here, however, we address the implications of interacting with a parent who is in no way physically maltreating, but—as a result of their own traumatic experiences or frightening ideation—sporadically alarms the infant via the exhibition of frightened, dissociated, or anomalous forms of threatening behavior. We suggest that spurious but ongoing interactions of this kind can occur even when a parent is normally sensitive and responsive to the infant, and can lead in turn to the infant's inability to remain organized under stress.

Many clinicians will no doubt have encountered cases in which they have determined that traumatic experiences on the part of the patient's *parents* have somehow indirectly become associated with the patient's own symptomatology, a conclusion which appears especially intriguing where it is otherwise difficult to convincingly identify more direct experiential origins of the patient's mental state. Findings that ultimately bear upon this particular kind of second-generation effect were first provided by these authors (Main and Hesse, 1990, 1992), and have been replicated in numerous investigations of other low-risk samples (see especially Ainsworth and Eichberg, 1991; van IJzendoorn, 1995; Hesse, 1999b). In these studies, the parent's unresolved/traumatized state has been identified via marked *lapses in the monitoring of reasoning or discourse* during the attempted discussion of potentially traumatic events within the Adult Attachment Interview. These lapses have repeatedly been found associated with an emerging marker of the increased likelihood of later mental difficulties, namely the infant's disorganized/disoriented behavior in Ainsworth's strange situation procedure (Ainsworth et al., 1978, discussed below). Recently, these "slips" in discourse or reasoning have been found associated with frightened and/or frightening interactions with the infant in the home or laboratory setting (Jacobvitz, Hazen and Riggs, 1997; Jacobvitz, 1998; Schuengel, van IJzendoorn and Bakermans-Kranenburg, 1997, 1999). In turn, frightened/frightening parental behavior as identified in the home, field, or laboratory setting has been found predictive of disorganized/disoriented infant strange situation behavior (Schuengel et al., 1997, 1999; True et al., 1998; Abrams and Rifkin, 1999; Lyons-Ruth, Bronfman, and Parsons, in press).

We begin this presentation with a review of relations emerging between disorganized/disoriented infant attachment status and varying kinds of later-developing psychological difficulty. For many children disorganized with the primary caregiver in infancy, these unfavorable sequelae include role-inverting (controlling) behavior toward the parent, representational and behavioral indices of continuing experiences of fear and anxiety, and several of the traditional indices of psychopathology. We then provide an overview of attachment theory, showing how being frightened by the parent places the attached infant in an irresolvable, disorganizing and disorienting paradox in which impulses to approach the parent as the infant's "haven of safety" will inevitably conflict with impulses to flee from the parent as a source of alarm. Here, we argue that conditions of this kind place the infant in a situation involving *fright without solution*, resulting in a collapse of behavioral and attentional strategies. In the succeeding sections, we clarify the inter-connections among the central phenomena, and describe each of the phenomena in greater detail. These include (1) the nature of disorganized infant strange situation behavior, (2) the nature of parental "slips" in reasoning and discourse surrounding the discussion of potentially traumatic experiences as observed in the Adult Attachment Interview, and (3) some of the associated anomalous forms of frightened and frightening parental behavior now being observed in both the home and laboratory. In conjunction with this latter description, we elaborate upon some of the intricate ways in which, for example, a frightened or dissociated parent can (like a directly threatening parent) place an attached infant in a paradoxical conflict leading to disorganization. The observations discussed originate primarily from the study of low-risk samples.

As implied earlier, our presentation may be of special relevance to those working with individuals (a) suffering from clinical levels of distress who (b) nonetheless evidence no clear history of either emotional or physical maltreatment, or indeed any other notable experiences of trauma. We suggest that in some such cases the patient's distress may represent a second-generation effect of their *parents'* own unresolved frightening experiences. Like their parents these patients will, however, also have been placed in confusing and frightening (albeit perhaps more subtle) situations, beginning in many cases at a far younger age.

Disorganized Attachment Status in Infancy and Middle Childhood: Relations to Psychopathology, Role-Inversion, and Continuing Indices of Fear

The Ainsworth strange situation is a structured observational procedure in which one-year-old infants are twice briefly separated from, and twice reunited with, the parent in a pleasant but unfamiliar laboratory environment (Ainsworth et al., 1978). Infants are categorized as disorganized/disoriented during the strange situation when they exhibit any of a wide variety of odd, inexplicable, conflicted or apprehensive behaviors in the parent's presence, such as leaning sobbing with head on wall and gaze averted, interrupting an approach to the parent by falling huddled to the floor, or freezing all movement with a trancelike expression (Main and Solomon, 1990). Despite the overtly unusual nature of many of these behaviors, a meta-analytic overview of studies of neurologically normal samples has strongly suggested that, within such samples, researchers should look to the infant's experience with the particular parent with whom the infant has been observed to be disorganized in order to provide an account for the appearance of these behaviors under stress. Thus, across studies there is to date no indication of the presence of a temperamental or constitutional component in disorganized strange situation responses (van IJzendoorn, Schuengel, and Bakermans-Kranenburg, 1999). Relatedly, infants generally exhibit disorganized behavior in the presence of only one of the two parents.

Unlike the three "organized" strange situation categories originally identified by Ainsworth (one secure and two insecure), disorganized/ disoriented strange situation behavior has been found predictive of psychopathology from middle childhood to late adolescence. Disorganized attachment status has repeatedly been found associated with unusual levels of aggression (i.e., disruptive/ aggressive or "externalizing" disorders) in both high-risk and low-risk samples (see Lyons-Ruth, 1996, for a narrative overview; see van IJzendoorn et al., in press, for a meta-analysis of these studies), and with internalizing disorders as well (for example, Moss et al., 1996; Moss et al., 1998). Additionally, using Sroufe and Egeland's large, high-risk sample of Minnesota 17-year-olds, Carlson (1998) found *overall* psychopathology as assessed by the K-SADS-E diagnostic interview (Orvaschel et al., 1982) substantially predictable from disorganized strange situation behavior with the mother during infancy. In keeping with a proposal advanced by Liotti (1992; see also Main and Hesse, 1992, Main and Morgan, 1996), Carlson (1998) also found infant disorganization in this sample associated with dissociative behavior as observed in the elementary school and high-school setting, and with dissociative experiences as assessed in the K-SADS-E interview at 17 years. Disorganization with the mother was also related to self-reported dissociative experiences at age 19, especially in cases of intervening trauma (Ogawa et al., 1997; the self-report inventory utilized was designed by Carlson and Putnam, 1993).

Infant disorganized attachment has, then, recently been linked with specific child and adolescent diagnostic categories. In addition, in the low-risk middle-class sample of Bay Area families studied by Main and her colleagues (Main, Kaplan and Cassidy, 1985) disorganized (as opposed to secure, avoidant, or ambivalent) attachment status in infancy had already been found to predict role-inversion with the parent in many children by age six, as well as response inhibition, disorganized and dysfluent discourse, and catastrophic fantasies. For example, in conjunction with this original study, Main and Cassidy (1988) reported that, when reunited with their parents following a one-hour separation, children previously disorganized with a particular parent were now controlling of (hence, role-inverting with) that same parent. Some of these children harshly ordered the parent about ("Sit down! I said, sit down!") or humiliated the parent by remaining silent in the face of the parent's overtures, comments or queries—behavioral responses termed *Controlling-punitive*. Others inverted roles with the parent by being excessively solicitous or caregiving ("Did you have a nice time while you were gone? Would you like to sit down and have me bring you something?"). These responses were termed *Controlling-caregiving* (Main and Cassidy, 1988). The development of *D-*

Controlling behavior at age six in children judged disorganized with the same parent during infancy has been replicated in three further studies (Wartner et al., 1994; Jacobsen et al., 1997 [see also Jacobsen et al., 1992]; and Steele, Steele and Fonagy, 1996). Indeed, the development of a controlling, role-inverting response to reunion with the parent with whom the child had been disorganized during infancy is sufficiently predictable that D-Controlling behavior is now used to identify disorganization in later childhood (van IJzendoorn et al., 1999).

Viewed at the *behavioral* level, then, early disorganization could seem to have disappeared by middle childhood, being replaced by organized (albeit controlling) behavior toward the parent. However, when asked to respond to imagined child-parent separations states of fear and mental or linguistic disorganization and disorientation have been found to persist (Kaplan, 1987; see also Main et al., 1985). Using an adaptation of Hansburg's (1972) Separation Anxiety Test (Klagsbrun and Bowlby, 1976), Kaplan reported that the majority of six-year-olds who had shown disorganized/disoriented behavior in the strange situation with the mother in infancy now demonstrated signs of being *"inexplicably afraid and unable to do anything about it"* (Kaplan, 1987, p. 109). As a series of six pictures involving separations ranging from a goodnight kiss, to the parents going out for the evening, to a two-week parental leave-taking was presented, the child was asked what he or she thought the pictured child would do, and how the child might feel. Overall, Kaplan identified the previously disorganized six-year-olds as *Fearful-Disorganized/disoriented* (hereafter, *D-fearful*). The central patterns which Kaplan considered indicative of continuing states of fear, disorganization, and disorientation are presented here in synopsis:

(a) *Direct descriptions of fearful events.* These included markedly catastrophic fantasies, such as suggestions that family members might come to great bodily harm, or even that the parents or child would die. For example, asked what the pictured child would *feel* one previously disorganized child (who had had no loss experiences) said:

She's afraid.
(Why is she afraid?)

Her dad might die and then she'll be by herself.
(Why is she afraid of that?)
Because her mom died and if her mom died, she thinks that her
    dad might die.

Asked what the pictured child would *do*, another previously disorganized child with no personal loss experiences responded:

Probably gonna lock himself up.
(Lock himself up?)
Yeah, probably in his closet.
(Then what will he do?)
Probably kill himself.
                        —Kaplan, 1987, pp. 109–110.

Other investigators have also noted the chaotic, flooded, catastrophic
quality seen in the responses to doll-play separations observed in
some disorganized children (Solomon, George, and DeJong, 1995). A
quotation from one D-Controlling six-year-old responding to a query
regarding what might happen during an overnight parent-child
separation may further clarify the frightening fantasies observed in
some children (Solomon and George, 1999, p. 17):

"And see, and then, you know what happens? Their whole house
blows up. See . . . they get destroyed and not even their bones are
left. Nobody can even get their bones. Look. I'm jumping on a
rock. This rock feels rocky. Aahh! Guess what? the hills are
alive, the hills are shakin' and shakin'. Because the hills are
alive. Uh huh. The hills are alive. Ohh! I fall smack off a hill.
And got blowed up in an explosion. And then the rocks tumbled
down and smashed everyone. And they all died."

(b) *Voicelessness and resistance*. These indications of a continuing
state of fear and disorientation were observed when a child suddenly
fell silent, began whispering, refused the task, or appeared too
distressed to complete it.

(c) *Disorganization in language or behavior*. This was observed in
children who responded to the pictured parent-child separations by

suddenly using nonsense language ("yes-no-yes-no-yes-no-yes-no"), making overtly contradictory statements without acknowledging the contradiction, or becoming behaviorally disorganized. For example, asked how the pictured child would feel, one child responded:

Happy.
(What's he happy about?)
'Cause he likes his grandfather coming. (Child jumps on back of stuffed animal in the playroom and hits it.) Bad lion! (Hits it more). Bad lion!
—Kaplan, 1987, pp. 110–111.

The association between the *D-Fearful* responses described above and early disorganized attachment status was marked, and Kaplan suggested that, because many of the disorganized children in the Bay Area sample had parents (termed *unresolved/ disorganized*) who still suffered from frightening ideation with respect to their own loss experiences, queries regarding separation might have had a particularly disorganizing effect on their children. In essence, Kaplan was proposing that the children's fearful fantasies, silences, and disorganized language or behavior regarding parent-child separations may have resulted from repeated interactions with parents who were themselves still fearful and confused regarding an important loss.

The association between infant disorganized attachment status and Kaplan's *D-Fearful* responses to separation pictures at ages six or seven has been replicated in Berlin (Jacobsen et al, 1997; Jacobsen and Hofmann, 1997; see also Jacobsen, Edelstein, and Hofmann, 1994). Similarly, using doll-play separations rather than separation pictures, Solomon, George and DeJong (1995) found that D-Controlling children fell in a response category similar to Kaplan's and termed *D-Frightened*, which included frightening stories (above), as well as response inhibition. A London study employing doll play with six-year-olds also found themes of violence, hurt, and illness significantly associated with infant disorganized attachment status with the mother during infancy (Steele et al., 1995).

Further indications of continuing fear specific to previously disorganized children in the Bay Area sample included frightening or frightened images and scratched-out figures observed in family drawings (Kaplan and Main, 1986), and dysfluent discourse with the parent on reunion (Strage and Main, 1985; see Main, 1995 for overview). In addition, Jacobsen (Jacobsen et al., 1994) found *D-Fearful* seven-year-olds in a large Icelandic sample had negative feelings about themselves, and (perhaps due to anxiety) exhibited marked difficulties in drawing the correct deductions in response to verbally administered reasoning tasks in adolescence. Finally, a post-strange situation rise in salivary adrenocortisal (a physiological index of stress) was found in disorganized infants in two independent studies (Spangler and Grossmann, 1993; Hertsgaard et al., 1995).

The relevance of the above findings to clinicians working with infants and children is clear. However, this presentation may additionally be of special interest to those working with older individuals whose early experiences do not appear to have been notably malignant or traumatic. Thus during therapy the offspring of a traumatized but non-maltreating caregiver might be expected to exhibit difficulties consonant with the sequelae to early disorganization described above, although these difficulties (see the prologue to this volume) may be the result of cumulative trauma as opposed to overt abuse. As adult patients, then, some individuals disorganized with one or both caregivers during infancy may suffer from recurring catastrophic fantasies, cognitive confusion, and blank spells; fall inexplicably silent for long periods; or attempt to control the clinician at times by becoming punitive or inappropriately solicitous.

One highly specific but particularly interesting possible sequela to early disorganized attachment status (drawn to our attention by Blatt and Diamond, personal communication, 1998) is a "fear of breakdown" as seen in individuals who have no remembered experience of a breakdown of any kind (Winnicott, 1974). In essence, Winnicott had argued that such fears regarding the future might in fact unconsciously represent fears of the return of an "original agony" (including what Winnicott had termed an "unintegrated state"), *which had in fact already occurred.* Elsewhere we have argued that repeated entrance into disorganized/disoriented states in infancy could have represented a kind of breakdown for some patients, particularly if extreme and arising as a result of frightening interactions with the parent. Thus, early disorganized attachment status could increase the risk for fear of breakdown (Hesse and Main, in press).

The discovery of disorganized attachment is embedded in a complex theoretical and empirical background. To understand the category, its correlates, and its implications for psychopathology, therefore, an orientation to the field is a necessity. For this reason, we next provide an overview of attachment theory emphasizing the evolutionary links between attachment behavior, fear, and survival. We then discuss research into parent-infant interaction which is currently being pioneered from within this context. We describe the surprisingly alarming behaviors associated with language and reasoning slippages surrounding the attempted discussion of traumatic events within the AAI, and observed in the parents of disorganized infants.

The essential position taken here is that, so long as the infant is not directly frightened by the parent, insensitivity to infant signals and communications will lead only to an insecure-organized (avoidant or resistant/ambivalent) attachment to that parent (see Main, 1990). *Fear of the parent*, in contrast, is expected to lead to disorganized attachment, and under certain conditions to increased vulnerability to psychopathology (see also Hesse and Main, in press).

Overview and background: Ethological-evolutionary attachment theory and the "organized" categories of attachment

Attachment Theory: Evolutionary Links to Fear and Survival

The infant's gradually developing tendency to cry when selected persons depart, to attempt to follow these persons when possible, and to cling to them and otherwise show pleasure upon their return appears to be relatively universally recognized, and a number of theories have been put forward to explain these phenomena (for an overview, see Ainsworth, 1969). Initially, most such theories rested on the reasonable supposition that the infant's focus upon specific persons was acquired only as they became associated with the satisfaction of more basic instincts. Thus, it was assumed that the infant's often highly emotional expression of attachment to parental figures is a secondary outcome of the parent's role in providing for the infant's more fundamental or "primary" drives, for example, feeding and related sensual gratifications.

If it were actually the case that early affectional ties are secondary rather than primary, however, young children should readily adjust to separations from attachment figures so long as food and other satisfying experiences are provided (Ainsworth, 1969; Bowlby, 1969). Early observations seemed to indicate instead that caregiving figures are not readily exchangeable and that extended, stressful separations from primary caregivers between 18 months and 3 years could have notably unfavorable consequences (Robertson and Bowlby, 1952; later, Robertson and Robertson, 1971, reported that such consequences are most pronounced when no consistent alternative caregiving figure has been provided). These observations were compatible with several object relations theories that stressed the intrinsic import of the infant's earliest relationships independent of their association with more basic "drives" (see Fonagy, 1999, for overview). Object relations theories can, however, still be sharply differentiated from attachment theory in that these theories do not place the infant's concern with maintaining proximity to the parent within the paradigm of natural selection. It is only within this latter context that attachment can be understood to be directly tied to safety and survival, and hence to fear.

The central formulations of this new approach to understanding the nature of the child's tie to its mother—called "ethological-evolutionary attachment theory"—were developed over a period of approximately 30 years (e.g., Bowlby, 1958, 1969, 1988). In an early clinical paper Bowlby reported that many patients seen in a juvenile guidance clinic were affectionless, and that the "affectionless character" was associated with histories of parental deprivation and/or repeated parent-child separations (Bowlby, 1944). This suggested that continuity in early parenting experiences played a specific and critical role in the ability to form affectional ties, a supposition that was corroborated by the observations of numerous clinicians and social workers (see especially Spitz, 1946; Goldfarb, 1943, 1945; summarized in Bowlby, 1951).

The proposition that to thrive emotionally children need a close and continuous caregiving relationship called for a theoretical explanation apart from the then prevailing views that love of the mother is either derived from or confounded with sensuous oral gratification, or is dependent on secondary reinforcement (Bretherton, 1992). Additionally, despite the fact that many object relations theorists had emphasized the import and primacy of parent-infant interaction, a consistent and well-articulated motivational model was still needed to account for this position. Perhaps in part serendipitously, it was at this time that Bowlby was alerted to recent developments in the field of ethology where it was reasoned that species' behavior patterns, like species' morphology, are the product of selection pressures and assist in individual survival (Bretherton, 1992). The work of Konrad Lorenz was of particular import in demonstrating that social bond formation need not be tied to feeding.

Following a review of evolutionary theory and the nonhuman primate literature guided in large part by the behavioral biologist Robert Hinde (Bowlby, 1986; Bretherton, 1992), Bowlby gradually came to the conclusion that crying, clinging, following and other behaviors that become focused on selected persons over the first year of life are to be attributed to the working of an attachment "behavioral system" (formerly "instinct", see Bowlby, 1969, Main, 1999, p. 847) which had, among other systems, been incorporated into the behavioral repertoire of ground-living primates in response to evolutionary selection pressures. It was further proposed that the selection pressure responsible for attachment behavior was specifically protection from predation, making the attachment behavioral system equal in import to feeding and mating in the immediacy of its implications for the individual's survival and ultimate reproductive success (Bowlby, 1969). Maintaining proximity to or contact with protective older individuals (attachment figures) would, then, decrease the likelihood that a particular infant would be targeted for predation. In addition, should an attack occur, flight to an attachment figure as a haven of safety would greatly increase the chance of infant survival. More recently, maintenance of proximity has been understood to promote survival by additionally providing protection from starvation, unfavorable temperature changes, natural disasters, attacks by conspecifics, and the risk of separation from the group (Main, 1979b, 1981; Bowlby, 1988).

In sum, attachment behavior is now viewed as the central mechanism regulating infant safety, and maintenance of proximity to attachment figures is understood to be the *sine qua non* of primate infant survival (Hinde, 1974; Hrdy, 1999). In consequence, attachment behavior is presumed to stand first in the hierarchy of infant behavioral systems. This is because within the environment(s) in which the human primate evolved even brief separations from protective adults will often threaten infant survival in a matter of minutes, and certainly within hours. In contrast, a considerable period of time can be spent without engaging in exploration, play, or even feeding. For this reason, whether or not attachment behavior is displayed at a given time, the young attached individual must at some level continually attend to the *safety* versus threat implicit in current conditions (cf. Sandler, 1960), while simultaneously monitoring the location and accessibility of those attachment figures upon whom its survival depends.

With the above in mind it follows that, in serving to protect the individual from danger, the attachment system must necessarily be closely intertwined with the fear (or "escape") system.[2] The activation of either of these behavioral systems does not, however, inevitably lead to identical outcomes (Bowlby, 1969). For example, given certain conditions, fear-evoking situations may lead to a wide variety of behavioral responses, such as freezing, crouching, trembling, attacking, and taking cover. In addition, among numerous *place-dwelling* mammalian species, a den, burrow, or other fixed location—rather than the mother or another individual—is commonly sought in times of alarm.

Ground-living primates are, however, largely nomadic, and as a result of their continuous movement do not establish a fixed location as a source of protection. Unlike those mammals for whom a special *place* provides the haven of safety, for the primate infant *the attachment figure is the single "location" which must be sought under conditions of alarm* (Bowlby, 1958, 1969). At such times, fear will most often activate attachment behavior, and hence the attachment and fear systems will operate cohesively and in tandem.

As this review indicates, then, *the attachment figure is the developing individual's primary solution to experiences of fear*, and this is of central import to our understanding of the relation between

---

[2] For heuristic purposes, behavioral systems are presented here as though completely separate and independent of one another. Behavioral systems are in fact inter-connected in complex ways (see Hinde, 1966; Bowlby, 1969), but discussion of this topic is beyond the scope of this presentation.

attachment, development and psychopathology. This relation rests in part upon the fact that, under some conditions, attachment behavior and fear ("escape") behavior are incompatible, and here conflict will almost inevitably occur. As is discussed below, this is particularly likely when the attachment figure (who is the infant's biologically channeled haven of safety) also becomes the source of its alarm.

The "Organized" Categories of Infant Strange
Situation Behavior: Patterns of Attachment Observed
with Parents Who are Not Directly Frightening

With the aim of describing the ways in which the infant comes to organize its attachment behaviors with respect to selected persons in normal circumstances, Mary Ainsworth undertook systematic home observations of infant-mother interaction in the first year of life, initially in Uganda (Ainsworth, 1967) and later in Baltimore (26 dyads, Ainsworth, Bell and Stayton, 1971; Ainsworth et al., 1978). In conjunction with these studies, Ainsworth (and other researchers; see especially Schaffer and Emerson, 1964) discovered that specific or "focused" attachments can be observed in most infants by the third quarter of the first year of life, and appear to be based upon contingent social interactions. Moreover, infants were observed to develop attachments to non-related individuals, and even to those who did not participate in their primary care. For many infants, two or more attachment figures were eventually selected.

Ainsworth, like Bowlby (1969) expected that all infants but those raised in extremely anomalous circumstances would have formed an attachment sometime near the end of the first year of life. This given, the primary question to be asked regarding a normally raised toddler's parenting experience was not *whether* she or he had become attached, but *how the attachment to the primary caregiver(s) had become organized*. The infants of insensitive and even maltreating parents were expected to be as fully (or "strongly") attached as were the infants of sensitive and responsive parents (see, e.g., Crittenden and Ainsworth, 1989). However, the organization of the infant's attachment to a particular parent, and correspondingly, the circumstances in which attachment behavior would be displayed or else inhibited was expected to differ across dyads.

Although initially relying exclusively upon home observations, Ainsworth had already recognized differences in the organization of infant-mother attachment in Uganda. It was not until she combined her Baltimore home observations with a structured experimental procedure, however, that she emerged with her three final patterns or "organizations" of infant-mother attachment. In Baltimore, 26 infant-mother dyads were visited for four hours approximately every three weeks across the first year of life, and interactions were recorded in the form of extensive narrative records. At the end of the year, each dyad was seen in a 15 to 20 minute structured, laboratory-based separation and reunion procedure in which the parent twice leaves the infant (once in the company of a stranger, and once entirely alone) and twice returns. This procedure, now known as the Ainsworth strange situation, was designed to create several "natural clues to danger" (Bowlby, 1973, 1969), including (a) an unfamiliar setting (b) in which the attachment figure departs. In keeping with Bowlby's theory, Ainsworth anticipated that by the time of the second separation, all home-reared 12-month-old infants would exhibit attachment behavior such as calling and crying for the mother (Ainsworth, personal communication, 1998). Once the dyad was reunited, however, the mother's presence was expected to provide sufficient security to permit the infant to return to exploration and play.

While the first Baltimore infant observed in the strange situation behaved as Ainsworth had predicted all home-reared one-year-olds would, ultimately just 13 of the 23[3] responded as anticipated. These 13 infants showed signs of missing the parent on departure (usually, by crying), sought proximity or contact upon reunion (usually, seeking to be held at least briefly), and then, apparently reassured by the mother's continuing presence, returned to play. Infants who responded in this manner were termed "securely attached" (pattern B), and this behavioral pattern was found strongly related to maternal "sensitivity to infant signals and communications"[4] as observed independently in the home (Ainsworth et al, 1978; see DeWolff and van IJzendoorn,

---

[3] Due to illness and other factors, the records of only 23 of the 26 infants seen in these original strange situations were ultimately retained.

[4] Ainsworth's definition of sensitivity was complex, and involved (a) noting that a signal had occurred, (b) interpreting it accurately, and then (c) responding promptly and (d) appropriately.

1996 for a meta-analysis of existing studies; see also Pederson et al., 1998). In essence, the response pattern displayed by secure infants appeared related to a history of interaction with a mother who tended to be prompt and comforting in regard to infant expressions of distress. Thus, infants displaying the secure strange situation response pattern were observed to have repeatedly experienced what B. Vaughn (personal communication, 1986) has termed "distress-comfort sequences," in which the mother had promptly and competently provided solace when her infant expressed fear, pain, distress, hunger or loneliness. Not unexpectedly, these infants rarely cried during brief separations within the less stressful conditions of the home (Ainsworth et al., 1971).

Two different types of strange situation response were found in the ten remaining Baltimore infants. One group (N = 6) showed few or no signs of missing the mother on separation, often even when left entirely alone. When reunited, they actively ignored and avoided the mother, moving away, turning away, and, if picked up, leaning out of the mother's arms, indicating a wish to be put down. These infants were termed insecure-avoidant (Pattern A), and despite a striking absence of observable affect during the strange situation, later studies would find indications of considerable distress at the physiological level (Sroufe and Waters, 1977; Spangler and Grossmann, 1993). Avoidance was associated with maternal rejection of attachment behavior, as implied by remarks indicating regret about having had the infant, and via direct observation of aversion to tactual contact (Ainsworth et al., 1978; Main and Stadtman, 1981; see Main, 1995). Intriguingly, despite the fact that neither anxiety or anger were displayed within the strange situation, avoidant infants exhibited high levels of anxiety and anger in the home (Ainsworth et al, 1978; see also Main and Stadtman, 1981, and Pederson and Moran, 1996).

The behavior of Ainsworth's four remaining infants provided a mirror image to those termed insecure-avoidant. Throughout most or all of the procedure, these infants were distressed and appeared highly preoccupied with the mother, with many showing little or no interest in the toys or other aspects of the environment. Often exhibiting anger toward the mother, these infants were unable to settle upon reunion, and were termed insecure-resistant or, alternatively, insecure-ambivalent (Pattern C). Like avoidance, resistance was found related to maternal insensitivity to infant signals, and specifically to a tendency either to pervasively ignore the infant, or to interfere with the infant's activities. However, rather than rejecting infant attachment behavior, and hence seemingly attempting to encourage the development of a precocious independence, the mothers of Group C infants were observed to discourage the development of autonomy (see Cassidy and Berlin, 1994; see also Solomon, George, and Ivins, 1987). Each of the resistant/ambivalent infants exhibited considerable anxiety within the home.

In sum, all of the infants in Ainsworth's Baltimore study had unquestionably developed an attachment to the mother which was readily observable within the home (Ainsworth et al., 1978). However, the organization of that attachment had been found to (a) differ among infants (b) in systematic accordance with the way in which the mother had responded to the infant during the first year of life (Ainsworth, 1991; see also Main, 1995). For the majority of infants, as expected, the strange situation elicited *only* attachment and exploratory behavior. Among those placed under the long-term strain imposed by varying forms of maternal insensitivity, however, new response patterns had appeared, interfering either with the expression of attachment (avoidance) or with the infant's ability to free its attention from the parent and engage with the environment (resistance). In our view, nonetheless, simple insensitivity to infant signals—whether displayed in persistent rejection of attachment behavior or in neglect, interference, or a failure to encourage the development of autonomy—is unlikely in itself to be alarming (see also Main, 1990).

In later years, the world-wide proportions of infants judged secure, avoidant or resistant in strange situation studies have been found to be highly similar to those established in Ainsworth's original sample (van IJzendoorn and Kroonenberg, 1988), and strange situation response appears to be independent of sex and birth-order. Additionally, in several investigations of low-risk samples, attachment to the mother has been found stable to at least six years of age (Main and Cassidy, 1988; Jacobsen et al., 1992, 1997; Wartner et al., 1994; Ammaniti, Speranza and Candelori, 1996).

Simple stability of response to the same person, even if indicative of continuing emotional security with respect to that person, does not, however, tell us whether security of attachment to the mother influences emotional well-being in settings in which she is absent. Fortunately, this critical question has been addressed in a series of studies of a large, high-risk poverty sample pioneered by Sroufe, Egeland and their colleagues, which include extensive longitudinal observations of children in school and camp settings. Here, children who had been judged secure with mother during infancy were judged more ego-resilient, more popular with peers, more competent, and happier than formerly insecure children (Weinfield et al., 1999; see also Main, 1973, and Troy and Sroufe, 1987). In many samples, the individual infant's attachments to its mother and father were found independent (i.e., the same infant was secure with one parent, but insecure with the other), and a series of critical investigations have provided little support for the otherwise reasonable supposition that genetic factors might contribute substantially to the organization of the infant's attachment to the parent (Sroufe, 1985; van IJzendoorn et al., 1992; Vaughn and Bost, 1999; Main, in press; van IJzendoorn et al., in press).

Additionally, each of the organized categories of infant strange situation behavior has repeatedly been found predictable from parental discourse within the Adult Attachment Interview, a structured, hour-long procedure in which individuals are asked to describe and evaluate early attachment-related experiences and their effects upon personality and current functioning (George et al., 1984, 1985, 1996; Main, Kaplan and Cassidy, 1985; see Hesse, 1999a, for overview). The interview is transcribed verbatim and, utilizing a system developed by Main and Goldwyn (e.g., Main and Goldwyn, 1984, 1998), most transcripts in low-risk samples can be assigned to one of three "organized" categories or "states of mind with respect to attachment"—secure-autonomous, insecure-dismissing, and insecure-preoccupied.[5] These adult attachment categories appear to provide

---

[5] Transcripts are assigned to the secure-autonomous category when the speaker remains coherent, consistent, and collaborative throughout the interview, whether early life experiences were favorable or unfavorable. Dismissing and preoccupied speakers lack the attentional flexibility and coherence evidenced in secure speakers, with dismissing speakers being especially striking for their failure to provide adequate support for positive descriptions of early experience, and preoccupied speakers seeming so excessively involved in early experiences with parents as to fail to simultaneously monitor the discourse context (Hesse, 1996).

Table 1 AAI classifications and corresponding patterns of infant Strange Situation behavior.

ADULT STATE OF MIND WITH RESPECT TO ATTACHMENT	INFANT STRANGE SITUATION BEHAVIOR
Secure/Autonomous (F) Coherent, collaborative discourse. Valuing of attachment, but seems objective regarding any particular event/relationship. Description and evaluation of attachment-related experiences is consistent, whether experiences are favorable or un- favorable. Discourse does not notably violate any of Grice's maxims.	*Secure (B)* Explores room and toys with interest in pre-separation episodes. Shows signs of missing parent on separation, often crying by the second separation. Obvious preference for parent over stranger. Greets parent actively, usually initiating physical contact. Usually some contact-maintaining by second reunion, but then settles and returns to play.
Dismissing (Ds) Not coherent. Dismissing of attach- ment-related experiences and rela- tionships. Normalizing ("excellent, very normal mother"), with generalized representations of history unsup- ported or actively contradicted by episodes recounted. Thus, violating of Grice's maxim of quality. Transcripts also tend to be excessively brief, violating the maxim of quantity.	*Avoidant (A)* Fails to cry on separation from parent. Actively avoids and ignores parent on reunion, i.e., by moving away, turning away, or leaning out of arms when picked up. Little or no proximity or contact seeking, no distress, and no anger. Response to parent appears unemotional. Focuses on toys or environment throughout procedure.
Preoccupied (E) Not coherent. Preoccupied with or by past attachment relationships/expe- riences, speaker appears angry, passive, or fearful. Sentences often long, grammatically entangled or filled with vague usages ("dadadada", "and that"). Thus, violating of Grice's maxims of manner and relevance. Transcripts often excessively long, violating quantity.	*Resistant (C)* May be wary or distressed even prior to separation, with little exploration. Preoccupied with parent throughout procedure, may seem angry or passive. Fails to settle and take comfort in parent on reunion, and usually con- tinues to focus on parent and cry. Fails to return to exploration after reunion.
Unresolved/disorganized (U/d) During discussions of loss or abuse, individual shows striking lapse in the monitoring of reasoning or discourse. For example, individual may briefly indicate a dead person is believed still alive in the physical sense, or was killed by a childhood thought. Individual may lapse into prolonged	*Disorganized/disoriented (D)* The infant displays disorganized and/or disoriented behaviors in the parent's presence, suggesting a tem- porary collapse of behavioral strategy For example, the infant may freeze with a trancelike expression, hands in air; may rise at parent's entrance, then fall prone and huddled on the

Table 1 Continued

ADULT STATE OF MIND WITH RESPECT TO ATTACHMENT	INFANT STRANGE SITUATION BEHAVIOR
Unresolved/disorganized (U/d) (cont.) silence, or eulogistic speech. The speaker will ordinarily otherwise fit to Ds, E or F categories.	*Disorganized/disoriented (D)* (cont.) floor; or may cling while crying hard and leaning away with gaze averted. Infant will ordinarily otherwise fit to A, B or C categories.

Two-week training institutes in the analysis of both the organized and disorganized categories of infant strange situation behavior are taught yearly by Alan Sroufe and Elizabeth Carlson of the Institute of Child Development, University of Minnesota, Minneapolis, Minnesota, 55455.

Two-week training institutes in the analysis of the Adult Attachment Interview are held regularly by several certified trainers (Nino Dazzi, Deborah Jacobvitz, David Pederson and June Sroufe). A list of available AAI institutes can be obtained from the first author at address listed at the end of this article.

Note. Permission to reprint this table, taken from Hesse (1999a) has been obtained from The Guilford Press. Descriptions of the Adult Attachment Classification System are taken from Main, Kaplan and Cassidy (1985) and from Main and Goldwyn (1984–1998). Descriptions of infant ABC categories are taken from Ainsworth et al. (1978), and description of the infant D category is taken from Main and Solomon (1990). Information regarding a fifth, "cannot classify" category not described here but prominent in clinically distressed and violent samples is available in Hesse (1996).

discourse parallels to the three "organized" infant categories[6] of strange situation response, and an overview is provided in Table 1. Secure-autonomous parents have repeatedly been found highly likely to have secure infants, dismissing parents to have avoidant infants, and preoccupied parents to have ambivalent/resistant infants (see Hesse, 1999a and Main, in press; see also van IJzendoorn, 1995). As noted earlier, however, some speakers—while usually appearing to be acceptably organized elsewhere within the interview—manifest disorganization and/or disorientation in reasoning or discourse specifically in response to queries regarding potentially traumatic events. Remarkably, these linguistic "slippages" are predictive of disorganized/disoriented infant attachment status.

---

[6]In direct parallel to "unclassifiable" infant attachment status as identified by Main and Weston (1981), a few transcripts have insufficient overall organization to permit assignment to the dismissing, secure, or preoccupied categories. These are currently termed "cannot classify" (see Hesse, 1996).

Disorganized Infant Strange Situation Behavior

In 1986, Main and Solomon first published their directions for identifying a fourth, disorganized/disoriented category of infant strange situation behavior (Main and Solomon, 1986). This category emerged through the meeting of two branches of inquiry which involved (a) the direct observation of conflict behaviors in infants and toddlers (Main, 1973, 1979a; Main and Stadtman, 1981) and (b) the recognition that some infants seen in the strange situation were difficult or impossible to classify (e.g., Main and Weston, 1981; Egeland and Sroufe, 1981; Crittenden, 1985; Radke-Yarrow et al., 1985).

Drawing on descriptions of what ethologists term *conflict behaviors*—that is, behaviors believed to result from the simultaneous activation of incompatible systems (see, e.g., Hinde, 1966; Tinbergen, 1951)—the second author had begun to code conflict behaviors in the toddlers observed in her doctoral thesis by 1972, and by 1974 undertook a second investigation of conflict behaviors, this time focusing upon the narrative records from Ainsworth's Baltimore sample (see Main, 1973; Main and Stadtman, 1981). Finally, utilizing yet a third (Bay Area) sample, a scale assessing "disordered/disoriented" behaviors was developed (Main, 1979a; see Main and Solomon, 1990, pp. 154–155). This scale was used applied to a videotaped procedure in which one-year-old infants are exposed to an initially silent, unmoving masked "clown" in the parent's presence (Main and Weston, 1981; see Grossmann, 1997, for a description of some unfavorable sequelae to "disordered/disoriented" behavior observed in the Clown Session in a South German sample).

In conjunction with Main and Weston's (1981) study, it was also reported that approximately 13% of infants in their large Bay Area sample were *unclassifiable* within Ainsworth's traditional, tri-partite system. A comparison of infant response to the "clown session" and strange situation behavior involving the same parent one week following revealed that conflict behavior was rare among secure infants, and was most pronounced among infants judged unclassifiable (Main and Weston, 1981). Thus a notable albeit preliminary association between the exhibition of conflict behavior in a stressful situation and unclassifiability with respect to the strange situation procedure had been established.

With the aim of better understanding unclassifiable attachment status, Mary Main and Judith Solomon (formerly a biological graduate student specializing in the study of animal behavior) undertook a review of these anomalous strange situation videotapes (Main and Solomon, 1986, 1990). Rather than revealing any new organized patternings across the course of the strange situation, unclassifiable infants were again found to display a diverse array of inexplicable, odd, or overtly conflicted behaviors, this time within the strange situation procedure itself. One unclassifiable infant, for example, cried loudly while attempting to gain her mother's lap, then suddenly fell silent and stopped moving for several seconds. Others were observed, for example, approaching the parent with head averted; rocking on hands and knees following an abortive approach; moving away from the parent to the wall when apparently frightened by the stranger; screaming for the parent by the door upon separation, then moving silently away at reunion; raising hand to mouth in an apprehensive gesture immediately upon seeing the parent at the door when reunited; and while in an apparently good mood slowly swiping at the parent's face with a trancelike expression.

The most striking theme running through the behaviors observed in these infants was that of *disorganization*, or an observed contradiction in movement pattern corresponding to an inferred contradiction in intention or plan (Main and Solomon, 1990). The term *disorientation* was also used to describe behavior which, while not overtly disorganized, nonetheless indicated a lack of orientation to the present environment (such as immobilized behavior accompanied by a dazed expression).[7] Seven thematic headings were identified, as presented in Table 2.

Bouts of disorganized/disoriented behavior sufficient for assignment to the D (disorganized/disoriented) category are often surprisingly brief (not infrequently consisting in just one episode lasting 10 to 30 seconds). For example, an infant who froze inexplicably in a posture which required physical effort to maintain (e.g., with one hand partially extended) for 20 seconds or more would be placed in the

---

[7] Directions for judging infants as disorganized were developed and refined through repeated study of 200 infant strange situation videotapes designated "unclassifiable" within the original three-part system—half drawn from low-risk and half from high-risk and/or maltreatment samples.

Table 2 Disorganized/disoriented behavior observed during the strange situation.

Strange situation behavior is judged disorganized when it fits to one of the following thematic headings:

(1) *Sequential display of contradictory behavior patterns.* For example, the infant may dash crying to the door at parent entrance, then fall silent and turn away to the wall.

(2) *Simultaneous display of contradictory behavior patterns.* For example, the infant may approach with head averted, or lean sharply away while clinging and crying. Also, while smiling and in an apparent good mood the infant suddenly strike or claw at the parent's face.

(3) *Undirected, misdirected, incomplete and interrupted movements and expressions.* For example, the infant may turn and brightly greet the stranger at parent entrance, or move sobbing to the wall rather than the parent when distressed.

(4) *Stereotypies, asymmetrical movements, mis-timed movements and anomalous postures.* For example, the infant may rock hard on hands and knees immediately on reunion, greet the parent with a one-sided smile, or repeatedly raise arms straight forward at shoulder height, eyes closed.

(5) *Freezing, stilling, and slowed movements and expressions.* For example, the infant may move very slowly towards the parent, as though moving under water or against physical resistance. Or, the infant may freeze all movement for 20 seconds, hands in air.

(6) *Direct indices of apprehension regarding the parent.* For example, the infant may place hands to mouth at parent entrance with a frightened expression, or may back against the wall with a fearful smile.

(7) *Direct indices of disorganization and disorientation.* For example, the infant may wander about the room in a disorganized fashion, turning in circles. Or, immediately upon parent entrance the infant may turn and brightly greet the stranger, raising arms.

Note: The above descriptions of disorganized/disoriented infant strange situation behavior are adapted from Main and Solomon (1990). Disorganized/disoriented behavior is scored by instance on a 9-point scale, and infants scoring above a 5 are placed in the disorganized category.

disorganized category. In addition, the disorganized category is always assigned together with a best-fitting, alternate avoidant, secure, or resistant category (e.g., disorganized/avoidant or disorganized/secure).[8,9] This is because the second best-fitting category may

---

[8] Also, some infants are alternately unclassifiable or cannot classify.

[9] Acceptable levels of reliability and stability were established for the disorganized strange situation category in this and succeeding independent investigations, and, additionally, across studies no significant sex differences have been found (van IJzendoorn, Schuengel and Bakermans-Kranenburg, in press).

ultimately be related to differing sequelae—that is, disorganized/ secure infants may differ markedly from those who are disorganized/ insecure, as Lyons-Ruth in particular has demonstrated (see Lyons-Ruth, Alpern, and Repacholi, 1993; Lyons-Ruth, 1996; see Lyons-Ruth and Jacobvitz, 1999 for overview).

Disorganized behavior has also been observed in infants and older individuals who are neurologically atypical (Main and Solomon, 1990; see also Pipp-Siegel, Siegel, and Dean, in press), isolated, or simply overwhelmed or over-stimulated by repeated or extended separations (Heinecke and Westheimer, 1966; Roberton and Robertson, 1971; Main and Solomon, 1990; Solomon and George, 1999; see Hesse, 1999b for overview). In addition, disorganized behavior (particularly, stereotypies and "freezing") can result from pharmocological interventions (see Hesse, 1999b).

However, since—in keeping with the theorizing put forward within this presentation—disorganization can also arise as the product of conflicting behavioral tendencies (Hinde, 1966), it is not surprising that disorganized behavior has been observed in experimental settings in which toddlers are deliberately given conflicting signals (Volkmar and Siegel, 1979; Volkmar, Hoder and Siegel, 1980), subjected to abrupt and confusing changes in interactional behavior, or else exposed to "inescapable" situations involving, for example, shame or embarrassment (see Main and Solomon, 1990 and Hesse, 1999b). Disorganized behavior in the presence of a particular parent may also result from circumstances in the parent's life which lead to frightened behavior only temporarily (a case of this kind in which an otherwise secure parent had just had a life-threatening experience is discussed extensively by Ainsworth and Eichberg, 1991). Since conflict arising in these latter situations is, however, either the product of experimental procedures or presumed to be transient, a search for ongoing and potentially disorganizing aspects of parental behavior was undertaken.

As noted earlier, we have hypothesized that behavioral and attentional organization can normally be maintained within the strange situation only so long as the attachment figure—whether sensitive or insensitive to infant signals and communications—has not been a direct source of fright (Main and Hesse, 1990, 1992; Hesse and Main, in press). The capacity to remain organized should, however, ordinarily break down in the face of repeated exposure to the inherently highly conflictual situation in which the attachment figure has become alarming.

In keeping with this proposal, disorganized behavior has now been observed in the great majority (77%) of maltreated infants studied in the strange situation in two relatively large independent samples (Carlson et al., 1989; Lyons-Ruth et al., 1991; see van IJzendoorn, Schuengel, and Bakermans-Kranenburg, 1999, Table 5). It is never-theless still necessary to provide an account for the fact that 15% of infants observed in low-risk samples (N = 2104; van IJzendoorn et al., in press) are disorganized, and that in several studies the proportion of middle-class toddlers judged disorganized has ranged above 30% (e.g., Ainsworth and Eichberg, 1991). Further, direct maltreatment is unlikely to provide the predominant explanation for the fact that in a study of children of mothers suffering from anxiety disorders, 65% of offspring were found disorganized (Manassis, Bradley, Goldberg, Hood, and Swinson, 1994). While of course no one would argue that maltreatment is absent in low-risk samples, or that it might not occur in some parents with anxiety disorders, it would be highly unlikely that, for example, 65% of mothers suffering from anxiety disorders would also be maltreating.

These findings, then, leave open the question of what the parental correlates of disorganized attachment might ordinarily be in non-maltreating populations, and indeed how disorganization can arise under circumstances that do not involve directly threatening or maltreating parental behavior. Ultimately, we theorized that *fright-ened* and *dissociated* parental behavior could place the infant in a paradox similar to directly threatening parental behavior, and that behavior of this kind could be expected in individuals in low-risk samples who were still frightened, unresolved, and disoriented with respect to their own experiences of loss or abuse.

Unresolved/Disorganized Adult Attachment Status: Discourse/Reasongin Lapses Occurring During the Discussion of Potentially Traumatic Experiences

Initial albeit indirect support for the above line of reasoning was provided by our early investigation of the Bay Area upper-middle-class sample (Main and Hesse, 1990). Here we found a strong association between the infant's disorganized/ disoriented behavior during the strange situation as conducted with a given parent and *linguistic slippages* observed in that same parent's discussion of potentially traumatic events sufficient to warrant placement in the *unresolved/ disorganized* Adult Attachment Interview category (Main and Goldwyn, 1984, 1998; see Hesse, 1999a and Hesse and Main, in press, for overview). In this study, we reported that 91% of mothers identified as substantially unresolved on the basis of discourse/reasoning lapses during discussions of loss within the AAI had had disorganized infants five years earlier, while only 16% of mothers who had *experienced* a loss, but showed little or no indication of disorganized mental processes in discussing the loss, had had disorganized infants.

The first replication study was conducted by Ainsworth and Eichberg (1991), who established that, in a sample of 50 Charlottesville mothers, those who had simply *experienced* a loss were no more likely than other mothers to have disorganized infants. However, *all eight* mothers whose lapses in reasoning or discourse identified them as unresolved/disorganized with respect to loss had infants judged disorganized with them during the strange situation.

The Ainsworth and Eichberg study provided a particularly dramatic example of a lapse in the monitoring of reasoning in a high-functioning mother. Immediately upon being queried regarding loss experiences, she responded "Yes, there was a little man" and then began to cry. The person lost was an elderly man who had worked briefly for her parents when she was eight years old. Jokingly, he had asked her to marry him when she grew up, and she had replied "No, you'd be dead." Not long after this exchange, he had died unexpectedly of a brain hemorrhage. Crying, this mother told the interviewer that it was she who had killed him—"with one sentence" (Ainsworth and Eichberg, 1991, p. 175). This lapse in reasoning was left unmonitored, leading to placement in the unresolved/disorganized adult attachment category, and as expected the infant's strange situation behavior was highly disorganized. The reader should note

(a)   the existence of frightening ideation (having killed someone with a thought) in this mother,

(b)   whose loss experience would not normally otherwise have been considered traumatic.

By 1994, unresolved/disorganized parental attachment status had been found predictive of infant disorganized attachment in five further samples (summarized in van IJzendoorn, 1995). In four of these samples, the Adult Attachment Interview was administered *prior to the birth of the first child* and compared to infant strange situation response to the same parent 15 months later (Benoit and Parker, 1994; Fonagy, Steele, and Steele, 1991; Radojevic, 1992, 1994; Ward and Carlson, 1995; the latter is a high-risk sample).[10] Since then, six additional investigations of the relations between unresolved parental attachment status and disorganized infant attachment status have been conducted, with highly significant linkages being reported for a majority of these studies (Hesse, 1999b).

In sum, then, researchers have repeatedly observed that (1) isolated, brief *linguistic* indices of disorganization and disorientation in the parent's AAI occurring specifically in response to queries regarding loss or abuse experiences (the majority of *unresolved* AAI's are otherwise globally well organized), predict (2) usually brief bouts of *behavioral* disorganization and disorientation in the infant. An overview of this system of linguistic analysis is provided in Table 3.

Frightened/Frightening Behavior in Non-Maltreating Parents

The first step toward deriving the conclusion that disorganized behavior could result not only from direct physical abuse and maltreatment (i.e., as a *direct* effect of trauma) but also as a *second-generation effect* of more subtle forms of parental behavior mediated by a frightened mental state (Main and Hesse, 1990, 1992) consisted in a closer examination of the "unresolved" interview passages in which linguistic slippages had been identified. Here we noted that in many cases the interviewer's questions regarding a potentially traumatic event seemed to have sparked or induced a momentary but dramatic alteration in the speakers mental state.[11] Indeed, many of the

---

[10] Interestingly, the strength of the association is highly related to the amount of training researchers have had in assessing disorganized strange situation behavior (Van IJzendoorn, 1995).

[11] States of absorption and intrusions from secondary systems are compatible with Hilgard's analysis of hypnotic phenomena and trancelike states (Hilgard, 1977) and with Bowlby's analysis of a case of unresolved mourning in an adolescent girl ("Geraldine," see Bowlby, 1980).

Table 3 Identifying unresolved/disorganized attachment status within the Adult Attachment Interview: Lapses in the monitoring of discourse and reasoning.

Lapses in the monitoring of *discourse* may take the following forms, among others:

(a) Sudden changes in speech register (e.g., shifting from normal speaking patterns into eulogistic/funereal speech, as, "She was young, she was lovely, and she was torn from us by that most dreaded of diseases, tuberculosis");

(b) Falling silent for 100 seconds mid-sentence, then continuing on unrelated topic;

(c) Giving extreme attention to details surrounding a loss or other potentially traumatic experience inappropriate to the interview context (e.g., a 10-minute discussion involving minute details of a loss including time of day, furnishings of the room, and clothing worn to the funeral by each family member).

Lapses in the monitoring of *reasoning* may take the following forms, among others:

(a) Subtle indications that a deceased individual is believed simultaneously dead and alive in the physical (not religious or metaphysical) sense (e.g., "It was almost better when she died, because then *she could get on with being dead*, and I could get on with raising my family");

(b) Placement of the timing of a death at several widely separated periods (e.g. ages 9, 11, and 15 given for same loss experience at differing places in the interview);

(c) Indications that self was responsible for the death where no material cause was present (e.g., death caused by having thought something negative about a person near the time of their death);

(d) Claims to have been absent at the time of the death, juxtaposed with claims to having been present (e.g., stating regret at having been at home when other family members were present at a drowning, then later speaking as though the self had been present: "and we tried, but none of us could swim to her").

Note: The above examples of lapses in the monitoring of reasoning and discourse are taken from Main and Goldwyn, 1998.

more marked slippages suggested that the speaker was experiencing either (a) high levels of absorption involving events which had as yet failed to undergo normal processing or (b) intrusions from a secondary (normally dissociated) ideational system involving those experiences, which was incompatible with an ordinarily more prominent view regarding these same events (Main and Hesse, 1990, 1992). As Table 3 indicates, examples of absorption included unusual attention to detail surrounding the discussion of a loss, or a sudden shift to eulogistic (funereal) speech. Lapses in reasoning suggestive of intrusions from a secondary, incompatible belief system were also found—for example, in statements indicating that a deceased person was believed still alive in the physical (as opposed to metaphorical, metaphysical or religious) sense. It appeared reasonable to assume, then, that *similar state-shifts could occur in such individuals in the home as well as the interview setting,* being triggered by (a) spontaneous intrusions from alarming memories or ideation and/or (b) something in the environment idiosyncratically associated with those ideas or memories.

As early as 1990, then, a theory was evolving which could in principle explain how a parent's unintegrated or dissociated state, including any concomitant fears and fantasies, could become associated with disorganized behavior in the infant (Main and Hesse, 1990, 1992). Having entered such a state, the parent might be expected to exhibit (1) anomalous forms of frightening or threatening behavior; (2) frightened behavior; or, simply (3) overtly dissociated behavior. For reasons which we delineate shortly, each of these subcategories of parental behavior is expected to be immediately frightening. In addition, depending on the nature and intensity of their own traumatic experiences, some unresolved parents might also (4) exhibit sexualized behavior, (5) treat the infant deferentially, timidly or as a protector, or (6) exhibit disorganized/disoriented behavior of the kind more commonly observed in infancy. These latter behaviors, although not necessarily immediately frightening to the infant, would nonetheless be most likely to occur if the parent had entered an "altered" or dissociated state. In this case, the parent could well be expected to become directly frightening, frightened, or dissociative at other times.

The above considerations, of course, would require empirical testing, and this led to the development of a coding system for identifying these kinds of parental behaviors (hereafter termed FR behavior, Main and Hesse, 1992–1998). An overview of this system is presented in Table 4.

This coding system was intended to provide a systematic means for investigating the hypothesis that *frightened and dissociated* behavior, as well as certain kinds of threatening behavior would appear in unresolved/disorganized parents in low-risk samples, and, like directly abusive or maltreating behavior, would place an infant in a behavioral/attentional paradox leading to disorganization and disorientation.

The FR coding system has evolved through several editions across the past eight years and, as of this writing, a number of independent investigators have utilized varying editions or portions of this system

Table 4 Precis of the Six Central Categories of the System for Coding FR Behaviors.

Note: Exclude from consideration simple disciplinary actions, even if somewhat harsh, insensitive, or momentarily frightening (e.g., shouting, or slapping of hand), or accidents that momentarily frighten the infant (e.g., slipping and bumping infant's head on wall), so long as parent's state does not appear dissociative or anomalous (see text, pp.).

I.   *Direct indices of entrance into a dissociative state.* For example, parent suddenly completely "freezes" with eyes unmoving, half-lidded, despite nearby movement; parent addresses infant in an "altered" tone with simultaneous voicing and de-voicing ("haunted" sound, as is produced by elongating the sounds of *"Hi"*, *"huh"* or *"ah"* while pulling in on diaphragm).

II. *Threatening behavior inexplicable in origin and/or anomalous in form.* For example, in non-play contexts, stiff-legged "stalking" of infant on all fours in a hunting posture; exposure of canine tooth accompanied by hissing; deep growls directed at infant.

III. *Frightened behavior patterns inexplicable in origin and/or anomalous in form.* Sudden frightened look (fear mouth, exposure of whites of eyes) in absence of environmental change. Also, a quick, stammering, alarmed retreat indicating that the infant must not follow, or approaching infant apprehensively as a potentially dangerous object.

IV. *Timid/deferential (role-inverting) behavior.* For example, submissive to infant aggression, hands folded, head bowed, no effort to stop painful slapping, hitting or hair-pulling. Also, turning to the offspring as a haven of safety when alarmed.

V.   *Sexualized behavior toward infant.* For example, deep kissing of infant, exhibition or encouragement of sexualized caressing.

VI. *Disorganized/disoriented behaviors compatible with Main and Solomon's (1990) infant system.* For example, mis-timed movements, anomalous postures, approaching infant with head averted, or any observable "collapse of behavioral (caregiving) strategy", such as becoming motionless while infant is crying.

Note: Readers interested in a more complete description of this system should write to the first author at address listed at the end of this article. Training institutes in the identification and scoring of FR behavior are being planned.

in home or laboratory observations. Two large-scale studies have investigated the relation between unresolved/disorganized (maternal) attachment status and FR behavior as observed in mothers in the home. Working at Leiden University in the Netherlands, Schuengel and his colleagues videotaped 85 mothers and infants for approximately four hours across the course of two home visits (Schuengel, van IJzendoorn, and Bakermans-Kranenburg, 1997). Home behavior observations were made at 10.5 months, and no instructions were given to mothers to engage in any particular forms of interaction. An association between unresolved/disorganized attachment and maternal FR behavior was found, but only when the mother's alternative or "best-fitting" AAI classification (assessed when the infants were 12 months) was insecure (Schuengel et al., 1997; Schuengel et al., 1999). This suggested the possibility of a protective factor operating to inhibit the expression of FR behavior in unresolved mothers whose underlying adult attachment classification was secure (a study of couple interaction, and a study linking the AAI to assessments of psychopathology appear to provide further corroboration of this proposal, see Hesse, 1999a, for review).

In a study conducted at the University of Texas, Jacobvitz, Hazen and Riggs (1997; Jacobvitz, 1998) administered the AAI to 113 mothers prenatally. Here, mothers were required to feed their babies, play with them, and change their clothing on camera. In this more stressful procedure, *both* unresolved/secure and unresolved/insecure mothers were far more likely to exhibit FR behaviors, as compared to either secure or insecure mothers who were not unresolved (similar results are emerging in a study comparing parental AAI attachment status to frightening/frightening parental behavior in a Bay Area study, Abrams, 1999). However, there was a tendency for unresolved/secure mothers observed in the home in the Texas study to exhibit somewhat less FR behavior than did unresolved/insecure mothers (Lyons-Ruth and Jacobvitz, 1999).

Two investigators have also examined FR behavior directly within the strange situation. A first study conducted with a middle-class sample at the University of Regensburg in Germany yielded no significant association between maternal FR behavior and infant disorganized attachment. However, these mothers were described as doing very little throughout the strange situation procedure as a whole, and the coders had not had the benefit of observing videotaped examples of FR behavior (Buttner, Hieber, and Grossmann, 1997). A second strange situation study, in contrast, utilized a high-risk sample, and wider variation in maternal behavior was observed. Here, FR behavior (as well as disrupted maternal communication and with-drawal) was found associated with infant disorganization, and the parents of disorganized infants whose alternative best-fitting classifi-cations were secure differed in intriguing ways from those whose alternative best-fitting classification was insecure (Lyons-Ruth et al., in press).

Several investigators have also examined the relation between FR behavior in the home, field or laboratory, and infant disorganized attachment status as assessed in independent strange situations. In the Leiden study of 85 dyads mentioned above, FR behavior as observed in the home at 10.5 months was significantly predictive of disorga-nized attachment in strange situations conducted at 14 to 15 months of age (Schuengel et al, 1999). In addition, a study of village-living members of the Dogan ethnic group conducted in Mali, West Africa, found a simplified assessment of FR behavior, as recorded in the field or hut setting, significantly associated with disorganized attachment status; however, no association was found in a second sample consisting of town-living Dogan (True et al., 1998; the village mothers were generally believed to be living in high-risk circumstances, as compared to the town mothers).

Finally, a study of 50 infant-mother and 25 infant-father dyads (total N = 75) conducted by Abrams at Berkeley was the first to use the most recent (1998) version of the coding system (Abrams and Rifkin, 1999; this study forms part of Abrams' doctoral thesis, and the full coding system is available as an appendix to Hesse, 1999b). Here, parents and infants were video-taped in the laboratory in 18 minutes of free-play, but—to create an opportunity for observing infant obedi-ence—parents were instructed to keep the infant away from various locations and objects. Free play was followed by the 12-minute Clown Session (Main and Weston, 1981), and coders, scoring across the full 30 minutes of observation, were blind to strange situations conducted one week previously. The results comparing parental FR free play/Clown Session classifications to infant D strange situation classi-fications assessed one week earlier were very strong for both mother-infant dyads (82% agreement, Fisher's exact test = .0002) and father-infant dyads (88% agreement, Fisher's exact test = .002). Across the 75 dyads as a whole, there was 84% agreement between FR and D classifications (phi = .61). Sixty-five percent of the (17) parents of infants assigned to D as a primary classification were judged FR, and 33% of the (6) parents of infants assigned to D as a secondary or "alternate" classification were judged FR. In contrast, only 4% of the (52) parents of non-D infants. Of the 15 out of 75 parents assigned to the FR classification, 11 had been assigned to D as a primary, and 2 as a secondary (e.g., secure/alternate disorganized) strange situation classification. Thirteen out of the 15 infants of FR parents had, then, shown substantial indices of disorganization and disorientation during the strange situation.

Considered as a whole, these studies provide preliminary (albeit correlational) evidence for the hypothesis that FR behavior frequently mediates the relation between unresolved (adult) and disorganized (infant) attachment status. It should be noted (a) that FR behavior may be most likely to appear among parents in high-risk samples, or when parents are observed in stressful settings, and consequently that (b) it may be under these conditions that stronger relations to unresolved maternal attachment status and disorganized infant attachment status are likely to be found. In addition, stronger results may be reported by researchers trained via a review of FR behavior examples, and able to utilize more recent editions of the coding system.

Below, we provide a general description of frightening and frightened parental behaviors which are *not* expected to produce disorganization. The behaviors found in the six categories of the FR system presented in Table 4 are then discussed, and illustrative case examples are given. In addition, we consider the ways in which each type of FR behavior may be directly (categories 1 to 3) or indirectly (categories 4 to 6) frightening and/or disorganizing to the offspring. It should be remembered that in all studies (other than the original study by Main and Hesse, which focused upon non-blind anecdotal observations), the observers of parental behavior have been blind to both the Adult Attachment Interview and infant strange situation behavior.

Frightened and Threatening Parental Behaviors
Not *Expected to Produce Disorganization*

In contrast to maltreating parental behavior, which must invariably arise from pathological conditions, there are several forms of frightened and threatening parental behavior that occur relatively frequently but would not normally be expected to lead to disorganization and/or disorientation. For example, Campos and his colleagues have demonstrated that infants as young as 11 months are highly alert to frightened expressions on the part of the parent which indicate danger. In Campos' studies infants have, for example, been observed to monitor and respond to parental expressions of apprehension or alarm as the infant approaches an apparently dangerous situation involving a simulated or "visual" cliff, and to inhibit movement across the cliff in response to fearful expressions (see Klinnert et al., 1983; Kermoian and Campos, 1988). Fearful parental expressions also, of course, appear outside of the laboratory setting, perhaps indicating approaching danger (e.g., the appearance of a potentially aggressive animal), or the possibility that the infant's actions may have immediately dangerous consequences (e.g., the toddler's movement towards oncoming traffic). In circumstances such as these, however, what is alarming— i.c., the source of the alarm—is *external* to the parent. The alarming stimulus will therefore ordinarily be both discernible and comprehensible, as will be made obvious in the parent's orientation, and the infant will be free to approach the parent. Moreover, it should be noted that when most parents themselves accidentally do something to frighten the infant, they are likely to immediately provide comfort, contact, or (in clinical terms) "repair" (see especially Lyons-Ruth and Jacobvitz, 1999, and Lyons-Ruth et al., in press).

Consider in addition the ordinary contexts in which threatening parental behavior arises. It is not unusual for a parent to become angry and/or threatening in disciplinary interactions—for example, when the child runs out into the street, or touches a forbidden object. At such times, the parent may not only sharply raise their voice, but also spank the child, or slap the child's hand. Here again, however, the stimulus for the parent's behavior is external and readily comprehensible. In addition, by changing its behavior via compliance, the offspring can in principle bring "frightening" parental behavior to an end. Finally, the child is often immediately able to (or even encouraged to) approach the parent, since the ultimate aim of such interactions is often protective, and this too provides an opportunity for "repair." Ordinarily, then, harsh or angry parental behavior in itself should not create an approach-flight paradox.

In sum, in the situations described above the conditions leading to parental expressions of fright or threat are discernible and comprehensible, while the expressions themselves are not anomalous. As a rule, it would therefore seem that circumstances of this kind should not interfere with the continued organized functioning of the attachment system.

Parental Behavior Likely to be Directly and Immediately Frightening and Disorganizing: Dissociative Behavior, Anomalous Threat, and Anomalous Expressions of Fright

Parental behaviors which are mediated primarily by internal factors related to unresolved experiences of trauma and fear will in general not allow for the regulated functioning of the child's attachment behavioral system. This will be likely because the parent's psychological state should most often be "altered" when these behaviors occur. The behaviors themselves can be delineated as follows.

Dissociated Parental Behavior

The phenomena of dissociation have fascinated clinicians and academicians since the early writings of Breuer and Freud (1895), as well as James (1890), Janet (1907), and Prince (1905). Especially careful descriptions and considerations of the phenomena of dissociation have recently been made available via the work of Hilgard (1977), Kihlstrom (1997), Liotti (1992, 1993, 1999), Putnam (1985), and Spiegel (1990), among others, although Ellenberger (1970) has pointed out that states of dissociation have a long history in human cultures.

Some aspects of dissociative experiences are subjective, and are therefore difficult to identify without direct query. These include depersonalization, amnesia, and the subjective sense of the existence of alternative identity states. Other arguably dissociative phenomena are, in contrast, clearly observable, such as trance states, and altered, anomalous facial and vocal expressions. As most readers are aware, the extremes of dissociative phenomena, such as dissociative identity disorder and fugue states, have frequently been associated with a history of trauma, and hence with fear (Putnam, 1985).

Dissociative parental behaviors were first found informally related to disorganized infant attachment status by Main and Hesse (1990) who, for example, described the simultaneous voicing and devoicing intonation used by some parents in greeting their (disorganized) infants. This intonation most often has a haunted or "Halloween" quality, not unlike that common to characters observed in "horror" films (as when "Hi . . . iiiii" is spoken while pulling in on the diaphragm). In a case seemingly also involving a dissociative element, a mother who had suffered abuse by her father was observed greeting her disorganized male infant with a sudden mid-sentence drop in intonation to a deep pitch more appropriate to a male. Like the de-voiced "*hi . . . iii*" described above, this vocalization struck listeners as markedly frightening, seeming "disconnected" from the mother's regular voice, and suggestive of intrusion from the voice of a second speaker. In more recent observations, one mother of a disorganized infant used a de-voiced whisper ("*aaaaau . . . ahhh,* get the blocks") in addressing her infant. This mother was also observed whispering instructions to herself just prior to speaking the same words in a normal conversational tone (Abrams and Rifkin, 1999). Remarkably, the voice heard as the mother almost inaudibly "coached" herself on how to act had the de-voiced or "haunted" quality described earlier. Another mother of a disorganized infant grunted and growled in a deep, aggressive and almost "inhuman" male voice while smiling and apparently pleasantly attempting to engage her infant in play. Each of these vocalizations was described as chilling and/or frightening when played for listeners, and suggested "possession" to one.

Another behavior pattern indicative of entrance into a dissociative state consists in "freezing" of all movement accompanied by half-closed, unblinking eyes. In such instances the parent appears completely unresponsive to, or even unaware of, the immediate external environment, including the movements and vocalizations of their infant. We have ourselves seen several unresolved/disorganized parents freeze all movement in the manner just described, while recently Jacobvitz (see Lyons-Ruth and Jacobvitz, 1999) has described her observations of one unresolved/disorganized mother who appeared to enter a trance state while being filmed in a feeding interaction in the home. Specifically, this mother sat immobilized in an uncomfortable position with hand in air, blankly staring into space for 50 consecutive seconds. In total, she entered apparently altered states for 5 out of the 20 minutes of feeding.

Dissociative or trance-like behavior this pronounced is rare in low-risk samples, and would be expected to receive the highest possible score (9 on the 1 to 9 point scale). Of course, more moderate examples of dissociative or dissociative-like phenomena are frequently observed, and receive much lower scores . For example, a mother may simply sit comfortably, maintaining a blank "unseeing" stare for a brief period while her infant moves about in front of her, vocalizing. In addition, fleeting, moderately "eerie" facial expressions have been noted in some mothers (see for example Schuengel et al., 1997).

It appears probable, however, that at high levels of intensity and/or in stressful situations, dissociated parental behavior can in itself be sufficiently alarming to leave the infant without a strategy for maintaining behavioral and attentional organization. For example, in three separate instances in which a parent used devoicing ("haunted") tones in addressing the infant, the infant's behavior immediately became disorganized. Similarly, two infants seen in the strange situation immediately "froze" (Main and Solomon's [1990] guidelines identify freezing and stilling as forms of disorganized/disoriented behavior) as soon as the parent entered into a trancelike state. When marked, then, many types of dissociative behavior are likely to be frightening. At the same time, in leaving the infant with "nowhere to go" (since the parent is visibly "not there"), a state of fright without solution will be created.

The existence of a specific and significant association between this (dissociative) subtype of FR behavior and infant disorganization was first uncovered in the Leiden study of infant-mother interaction in the home described above (Schuengel et al., 1997). A very strong relation between FR scores assigned specifically for dissociative behavior and the degree to which the infant had shown disorganization with the same parent was also found for both mother (N = 50, r = .49) and fathers (N = 25, r = .48) in the Bay Area study (Abrams and Rifkin, 1999). Because for reasons not yet known mildly dissociative behaviors, such as trancelike stilling, seem to occur more frequently in low-risk samples than the anomalous forms of threatening and frightened behavior described directly below, it is likely that this particular subtype of FR behavior will continue to show a strong relation to unresolved parental and disorganized infant attachment status.

Anomalous Forms of Threatening Parental Behavior

As early as 1990, Main and Hesse had called attention to some unusual parental movement patterns observed during the strange situation with disorganized infants. These included startling, unpredictable invasions of "personal space"—for example, while seated behind the infant, some parents silently and suddenly slid their hands across the infant's face or throat. In addition, we informally noted non-gamelike movements or postures that resembled a hunt or chase-pursuit sequence in the parents of some disorganized infants, almost as though the infant were being stalked.

Surprisingly, since our early non-blind observations of threatening and non-game-like "hunt-pursuit" sequences in a few parents seen in the strange situation, several independent researchers utilizing home or laboratory free play observations have reported the sudden appearance of predatory and/or animal-like forms of threatening behavior in the parents of disorganized infants. In some cases, these parents have simply been observed to abruptly begin to stalk the infant on all fours, silent and stiff-legged, in the absence of all "meta-signals" of play. In the study conducted at Leiden, for example, one unresolved mother of a disorganized infant suddenly crawled silent and catlike towards her infant and then, simulating "mauling" behavior, turned her over with fingers extended like claws (see Schuengel et al., 1997). This mother also combined tickling with baring her teeth and looming over the baby's face, increasing and continuing this display as the baby became frightened. Another unresolved mother of a disorganized infant clawed repeatedly toward her infant's face, while the mother of an unclassifiable infant[12] tossed her toddler in the air while growling and baring her teeth.

---

[12] As noted earlier, the identification of disorganized infant strange situation behavior evolved out of an examination of infants whose strange situation behavior was unclassifiable. Schuengel and his colleagues describe this infant's strange situation behavior as not only failing to fully fit to the traditional A, B, and C attachment categories, but to the D category as well (Schuengel et al, 1997). Our own (still informal) ongoing analyses of strange situation behavior are continuing to suggest that unclassifiable infant strange situation attachment status has correlates similar to that of disorganized attachment status.

Recent observations in the free-play laboratory context made by Abrams and Rifkin at Berkeley (1999), and home observations by Jacobvitz at Texas (Jacobvitz, 1998; see also Lyons-Ruth and Jacobvitz, 1999) have continued to confirm the existence of "predatory" forms of threat behavior in parents independently identified as having disorganized infants. These behaviors have included not only teeth-baring but, in addition, cat-like hissing, deep threatening growls, and even one-sided lip-raising (in essence, one-sided canine exposure, a threat gesture noted by Darwin in 1872) have been observed. None of these predatory behaviors and expressions appear to be playful, and most seem to arise "out of nowhere," and then disappear. However, since the attachment behavioral system is believed to have evolved primarily to protect the infant from predation (Bowlby, 1969), behaviors of this kind may be especially frightening and be expected to arouse the attachment system at the highest level of intensity.

The approach-flight conflict leading to disorganization within the context of (anomalous) threatening parental behavior should, of course, generally be the same as that described earlier for cases of battering. Because most of the anomalous forms of threatening behavior described above appear suddenly, briefly, and without apparent context, we infer that fleeting affects—including frightening, partially dissociated memories or thoughts associated with the parent's own trauma or fearful ideation—may drive the abrupt appearance and disappearance of these behaviors. It should be noted that in the Bay Area study of 50 infant-mother dyads described earlier (Abrams and Rifkin, 1999), scores for these anomalous (predatory) forms of maternal behavior were found in themselves significantly associated with infant disorganized behavior as assessed one week previously.

Anomalous Forms of Frightened Parental Behavior

We now turn to the more subtle and initially perplexing problem of why certain anomalous expressions of *fright* are also likely to lead to disorganization in the offspring. Ultimately, we believe that in this context the operative mechanism also involves alterations in normal consciousness originating from the parent's traumatized state of mind.

Here, however, rather than resulting in readily observable dissociative states or agonistic propensities, trauma and frightening ideation seem to have led to sporadic unintegrated expressions of fright.

Unlike anomalous threat, which may eventually be found associated with an underlying insecure (e.g., unresolved/dismissing or unresolved/preoccupied) state of mind on the part of the parent, there is no reason to assume that anomalous expressions of fright might not often occur in otherwise secure, and normally sensitive, parents. It is of special import, then, that in her study of parental behavior during the strange situation Lyons-Ruth (see Lyons-Ruth and Jacobvitz, 1999, p. 531) found that mothers of disorganized infants showing an underlying or "alternate" secure AAI response differed from the mothers of disorganized infants showing an underlying insecure patterning, in that the former exhibited *fearful-inhibited* behavior. Strikingly, then, the mothers of disorganized/secure infants were characterized as manifesting subtle, *frightened* behavior in the absence of high levels of frightening, dissociated or role-inverting behavior; in addition, they were sometimes described as withdrawn, without being hostile.

Below we identify and describe two anomalous forms of frightened behavior observed in the parents of disorganized infants: frightened behavior which has no evident environmental source, and behavior indicating that the parent is *frightened of* the infant. Again, as noted above, and as Lyons-Ruth's findings would suggest (Lyons-Ruth and Jacobvitz, 1999; Lyons-Ruth et al., in press), these behaviors are not necessarily incompatible with parenting which is otherwise relatively sensitive and responsive.

Anomalous Forms of Frightened Behavior Presumed to Occur
in Response to Environmental or Internal Events Associated
with the Parent's Unresolved State of Mind

Expressions of fright stemming from the parent's past experiences will most often ultimately be internal in origin, and therefore frequently unlocatable within the infant's immediate environment. Thus— whether triggered by an internal stimulus, or by some external stimulus idiosyncratcially associated with the parent's history or ideation— when such expressions are perceived the infant will "sense" impending danger, the source of which will be either indiscernible or incomprehensible.

Providing one example of behavior of this type, Main and Hesse (1990) described the parent of a disorganized toddler who responded with an immediate, frightened intake of breath as he began moving a toy car across the room, and then cried out "Uh-oh! Gonna have an *accident*! Everybody's gonna get *killed*!!" Although we had no access to this parent's history, the panic implied by the frightened intake of breath combined with the particular statement made could well suggest some connection to earlier personal or familial experiences of loss through automobile or other accidents. This is, of course, only one idiosyncratic example, while a parent who suddenly looks about or reacts to an unchanged benign environment with alarm provides a more general illustration. As another example, for no cause apparent to the offspring, a parent who had lost a family member through drowning could suddenly tighten his or her grip on the infant with an accompanying sharp intake of breath while friends discussed a trip to the seashore.

Parental behavior of this kind would almost inevitably be alarming, since it suggests an immediate (albeit indiscernible) danger. However, as in the case of dissociative states described earlier, a parent behaving in a frightened manner for these reasons is unlikely to appear sufficiently externally oriented to provide adequate protection. Indeed, although a parent engaged in an anomalous display of fright may not simultaneously appear to be in a dissociative state, the arousal of unintegrated fear will no doubt normally be the product of a somewhat altered state of consciousness. In some cases, the parent may simply sporadically enter general states of alarm, which stem from changes in unconscious factors that have no systematic relation to particular events or elements within the immediate environment. In other cases, the stimulus for the parent's alarm can be traced and defined but has no obvious or immediate link to danger (e.g., the previous reaction to discussions of trips to the seashore). As when the parent more obviously enters a dissociative state, then, the parent is likely to be both alarming and simultaneously unavailable, placing the infant in a situation involving fright without solution.

Frightened behavior indicating that the infant itself is the source of the parent's alarm. For a parent who remains frightened by partially dissociated experiences, a number of complex and confusing responses to the infant may arise, some of which will involve situations where the infant becomes confused or identified with the original experience or its associated ideation. Main and Hesse (1990) described one (unresolved/disorganized) parent backing away from their infant during the separation episode of the strange situation, while stammering in an unusual and frightened voice: "D-don't follow me, d-don't." During the succeeding reunion, the infant lay stilled and flattened against the parent with eyes dazed for over one full minute, and was judged disorganized. The mother of another disorganized infant was observed jerking her head away with a fear grimace and eyes wide, when the infant reached out to pat her face in a calm and exploratory manner. Intriguingly, frightened parental head movements have now been observed in several samples as the parent responds to the approach of the infant's hand. In addition, parents have been observed stepping cautiously from place to place as though attempting to keep the offspring at the greatest possible distance, or even attempting to "escape" the infant by moving out of reach as if the infant was, for example, a pursuing and potentially dangerous animal. Finally, the unresolved/disorganized mother described earlier as having entered trance states during a feeding interaction in the Texas study was also observed suddenly moving her hand away from her infant as if fearful of being hurt (see Lyons-Ruth and Jacobvitz, 1999).

How can we account for such anomalous responses to infants, who in fact have no direct power to harm? One among many possible explanatory pathways could involve experiences which, whether inherently traumatic or simply associated with frightening ideation, occurred when the parent was a child. Consequently, in some cases the offspring may become unconsciously confused with these experiences, leading to the "unprocessed" conclusion that the child is a source of alarm. Here the reader may recall that the unresolved mother of a disorganized infant discussed by Ainsworth and Eichberg (1991, above), appeared to retain the childhood belief that, at age eight, she had killed her caretaker "with one sentence!". If at certain moments such a speaker believes that children have the power to kill through thoughts or sentences, the correlated idea *that it is possible to be killed by one's own offspring* could then well arise. "Anniversary" reactions occurring when an offspring reaches the age at which the parent lost an important person may therefore not only be mediated by, for example, the renewed onset of depression, but also in some cases by the re-arousal of anxiety and fright. Fear *of the offspring* in traumatized parents is therefore perhaps not as unlikely an outcome as might be imagined, especially since some mothers describe their disorganized children as having supernatural powers, and special connections with deceased persons (see Solomon and George, 1999).

It should additionally be noted, however, that when the source of danger is thought by the parent to emanate specifically from within the infant, the infant's position becomes especially perplexing and disorganizing. Conceivably, it may lead the offspring to the following experiences, observations or suppositions, however inaccessible to consciousness and/or infantile in form:

(1)   Attempts to increase proximity to the parent are, paradoxically, likely to trigger parental inclinations (however subtle) to increase parent-offspring distance. Moreover, rather than appearing simply indifferent to (neglecting of) the infant, the retreating parent will often appear alarmed.

(2)   Over and above the fact that the attachment figure cannot be approached as a haven of safety (point 1), *there can be no escape from a source of danger which emanates from within the self*. More specifically, if the *offspring* is treated as an apparent source of danger, he or she is subjected to the additional frightening, paradoxical and disorganizing condition of *needing to take flight from the self*.[13] Main and Hesse (1992) have suggested that under extreme conditions one "solution" to the approach/flight paradox created by an alarming parent could be the "creation" of two selves or executors, one to approach, and one to take flight. Similarly, the ultimate "solution" to this even more perplexing situation (in which the self comes to be perceived as the source of danger) could involve the creation of segregated systems or multiple executors (selves, see Bowlby, 1980, Hilgard, 1977). Here, however, rather than simply needing two selves to perform contradictory actions, two selves are needed in order for one to retreat from the second. While

---

[13] This condition may await the development of a sense of self and cognitive abilities which appear shortly after infancy.

perhaps a rare outcome of such experiences, these circumstances provide a particularly compelling backdrop for "splitting" or dissociative sequelae in the event of future trauma.

(3)   Finally, as is known from observations of animals, flight behavior on the part of one individual can be a stimulus provoking attack or hunt-chase behavior on the part of a second (T. Johnson, personal communication, 1994). Therefore, like a cat who only arouses chase behavior in a dog if it takes flight, a parent who exhibits fear or inclinations to take flight in response to infant approach could provoke aggressive or "chase/pursuit" tendencies. Such conditions might gradually stimulate the development of inclinations to "attack" the parent, and con-tribute to the intensification of both frightening and aggressive ideation. Ironically, the more subtle the nature of the interaction, the more confusing and difficult the outcome might be for the offspring. Indeed, identifying the origin of intrusive, aggressive ideation resultant from interactions with a subtly frightened parent could be difficult for patient and clinician alike, unless both were alerted to investigate the patient's responses to fright-ened behavior in other persons.

In summary, within the context of dissociated parental behavior in general, and more specifically in circumstances where the parent exhibits anomalous forms of threatening or frightened behavior— including the special case in which the parent appears to be alarmed by the infant—several direct pathways to disorganization can be identified.

Other Forms of Behavior Likely to be Associated with
Unresolved Mental States in the Parent: Timid/deferential,
Sexualized, and Disorganized/disoriented Behavior

The behaviors which remain to be discussed comprise the final three of the six subcategories delineated in the FR coding system, and are now briefly reviewed. While these latter behaviors may in themselves be less likely to lead directly to an approach-flight paradox for the infant, they each imply the appearance of an alteration in normal consciousness on the part of the parent, which may increase the likeli-hood that the anomalous behaviors capable of directly producing disorganization may appear at other times.

Timid/deferential Behavior, and (Role-inverting) Tendencies
to Utilize the Offspring as an Attachment Figure in Times of
Distress or Alarm

In our original observations of the strange situation behavior of the
parents of disorganized infants, we described "extreme timidity" in
one mother's handling of her infant, while a second (unresolved/
disorganized) mother appeared timidly responsive to indications of
infant anger (Main and Hesse, 1990). The latter observation was made
during a reunion episode, in which the mother sat erect, welcoming
her approaching infant with extended hands. However, when her
daughter made an impatient gesture, the mother responded by slump-
ing her shoulders, folding her hands, and assuming an humble
"waiting" posture, accompanied by a pleading look. Similar timid/
deferential behavior was observed in the Dutch study (Schuengel et
al., 1997), in a mother assigned to the unresolved AAI category on the
basis of lapses in reasoning and discourse as she described her
mother's suicide. Several times, in response to infant noncompliance,
this mother retracted her hands and folded them before her chest with
her shoulders lowered and her gaze cast downward, as though
apologizing. Her infant's strange situation behavior was anomalous,
but did not quite meet the criteria for being categorized as disorganized. While these instances of timid/deferential parental behavior are
moderate, we have also noted more extreme examples, such as deferential submission to obviously painful slapping, hitting or hair-pulling.
In each of these more extreme cases, the infant was disorganized, or
else unclassifiable.

What the examples described above have in common is that the
parent appears to treat the infant as superior and/or as having greater
power. This observation accords with George and Solomon's (1996)
finding, noted earlier, that the parents of disorganized children sometimes consider the child to have supernatural capabilities, and that (as
identified from a caregiving interview) these parents feel helpless with
respect to their offspring who are, correspondingly, perceived as
powerful. Despite the fact that no direct evidence is as yet available,
we can also imagine that some parents who exhibit timid/deferential
behavior toward the infant during videotaped interactions may at other
times experience propensities *to seek the infant as a haven of safety*
when alarmed.

Since an infant in fact has no capacity to protect the parent, we may well ask how behavior of this type can arise. It should be recalled, however, that in ground-living nomadic primates at least two relatively universal tendencies are aroused in conjunction with heightened states of alarm.[14] The first is to take flight from the perceived source of danger, and the second is to seek the proximity of an attachment figure who provides protection at such times. In consequence, not only the infant *but the parent as well* should experience a volition to seek a haven of safety if sufficiently alarmed. In most parents, of course, any propensities to seek the offspring as a haven of safety are either absent or ordinarily over-ridden, so that alarm stemming from an environmental source most often elicits a protective, as opposed to a protection-seeking, response (Cassidy, 1999).

Some parents in unresolved mental states may at times nevertheless experience a disoriented volition to seek the offspring when alarmed. This anomalous inclination would no doubt be involuntary, and in some way intended to reduce parental fear. If acted upon, however— even simply as an observable momentary inclination—the infant's immediate confusion would almost inevitably be heightened.

In this case, the infant is not faced with the problem of a frightened, retreating parent, i.e., one who responds to approach behavior with propensities to increase distance. Nonetheless, if the parent is approaching the infant as a source of safety because they are in an alarmed state, an approach-flight paradox will still be created, since the source of the infant's alarm (the frightened, approaching parent) will still activate simultaneous inclinations to increase proximity as well as distance.

Sexualized Behavior

Overtly sexualized behavior towards infants is rarely observed in low-risk samples. However, mild forms of these behaviors do occur, as Abrams and Rifkin (1999) have recently observed in one parent of a disorganized infant who suddenly, but very briefly, grunted and twisted her body suggestively towards her infant with a "come-hither" expression. In a few samples, overly intimate kissing of the infant has been observed and/or the infant has been encouraged to engage in

---

[14]In older individuals, both the protective and agonistic systems may also become activated.

caresses that appear romantic in nature and elicit a dreamy or romantic look in the parent.

In all cases of sexualized/romanticized parental behavior noted to date, the infant's strange situation response has been either disorganized or unclassifiable. However, most of the sexualized behavior we have observed on videotape is engaged in by parents whose immediate appearance is neither frightening or frightened, nor (with some exceptions) overtly dissociated. Instead, the parent not infrequently seems gentle, affectionate, and pleasant, and the behavior appears to have no immediately frightening effect. However, it seems difficult to imagine that members of the particular westernized nations observed in these studies could (a) lack the ability to monitor their actions sufficiently to permit them to observed behaving in a markedly sexualized manner toward their infants without (b) having had experiences rendering them vulnerable to exhibiting overtly dissociated and even frightened or frightening behavior at other times.

Disorganized/disoriented Behaviors
Compatible with the Infant System

From the first, the FR system for identifying frightened/frightening parental behavior has included behaviors which had originally been identified as disorganized/disoriented in the infants originally studied by Main and Solomon (1986, 1990). However, following Liotti's (1992) suggestion that disorganized infants would be more vulnerable than others to develop dissociative disorders in later life, we had earlier reviewed the indices of disorganized/ disoriented strange situation behavior, finding that many such behaviors (e.g., trancelike stilling and freezing) appeared phenotypically dissociative (see Main and Morgan, 1996). Some "disorganized/disoriented" infant behaviors were therefore placed under the FR sub-heading of directly "dissociative" (parental) behavior. However, a separate sub-heading for "any [other] disorganized/disoriented behavior fitting to the infant system" was also included, and researchers working with the FR system were encouraged to look, for example, for asymmetrical expressions and mis-timed movements (Main and Hesse, 1992–1998).

To our knowledge it is only recently, however, that disorganized parental behaviors fitting to the principles of the *infant* system have actually been noted, and connected to infant disorganization. In their study observing infant-mother interaction in the Main and Weston

(1981) free play and Clown Session procedures, Abrams and Rifkin (1999) have noted two intriguing forms of disorganized/disoriented behavior in some parents of disorganized infants. For example, in keeping with the infant disorganized coding system, two mothers of disorganized infants suddenly appeared "blind" (both facially and by changes in movement pattern), whereas previously the functioning of their eyes had appeared normal. Another suddenly moved in a stiff, asymmetrical, robot-like manner suggestive of someone with neurological impairments or who was recovering from a severe injury. Assuming no momentary neurological interference (the mother moved normally at other times) her behavior was inexplicable, suggesting a momentary "collapse of behavioral strategy".

These findings regarding the varying subtypes of frightened/frightening parental behavior, as well as the broader sets of findings and results discussed earlier (e.g., Jacobvitz, 1998; Schuengel et al., 1997, 1999; Abrams and Rifkin, 1999; Lyons-Ruth and Jacobvitz, 1999; Lyons-Ruth et al., in press) suggest that observational research using the FR system will continue to yield new and intriguing information regarding these sporadic "lapses" in parental action. A task for the future will be to explore the possibility of linkages between specific kinds of discourse/reasoning lapses in the AAI, and particular subtypes of FR behavior. For example, it could be that the subject matter involved in the linguistic lapses (e.g., physical abuse as opposed to loss) is related to the subtypes of FR behavior which are displayed (e.g., anomalous forms of threatening behavior as opposed to dissociative behavior). Additionally, lapses in reasoning may be more commonly associated with a different cluster of FR sub-types than are lapses in discourse. Any systematic differences uncovered regarding the precursors of or sequelae to different FR interactions would of course be of great interest, but an investigation of this kind will no doubt have to await the collection of data from a large number of studies.

Summary and Conclusions

In this paper, we have identified a number of circumstances which should lead to the arousal of fear in the infant and specifically, fear of the parent. We have proposed that the infant repeatedly frightened by its parent does not merely experience negative and disturbing emotion(s), but additionally is subjected to a biologically channeled paradox in which simultaneous propensities to approach and to take flight from the parent are activated.

Many theories focusing upon early development would of course concur that parental behaviors which frighten the offspring will have untoward effects. It is specifically attachment theory, however, which posits that the biological function of the child's tie to its primary care-giver(s) is protection, and that among ground-living primates, the attachment figure provides the infant's primary solution to situations of fear (Bowlby, 1969). Attachment theory has, then, created the framework for the proposal that parental behavior which frightens the infant will drive the infant *towards* (as well as *away from*) the parent. It is via this paradox that a conflict capable of overwhelming the young infant is produced—a conflict which in turn frequently leads to disorganization and disorientation. In addition, we have proposed that the paradoxical situation created by fear of the parent may cause a lowering of attentional capacities and relatedly, temporarily restrict or alter the child's capacity for normal conscious processing. Alterations in consciousness in the face of an approach-flight paradox may, there-fore, be associated with difficulties in maintaining the capacity for normal information-processing. This proposition remains to be fully explored but may provide a useful point of entry for enhancing our understanding of the psychological vulnerabilities presently being found associated with early disorganized attachment (see Main and Hesse [1992] and Hesse [1999b] for a discussion of serial vs. parallel informational processing in this context).

Within this presentation, we have outlined a pathway from certain anomalous forms of parental behavior to a variety of unfavorable outcomes for the offspring which would otherwise have often appeared untraceable with respect to a direct experiential source. Earlier, by studying the lapses in the monitoring of discourse or reasoning which occurred as the parents of disorganized infants attempted to discuss loss or abuse experiences, we had discovered "parapraxes"[15] or slips in the parent's *language* which were predictive of parapraxes in the *infant's actions*. We presumed that these slips

---

[15]Readers outside of the analytic community may be less familiar with the term "parapraxis," indicating a "... faulty action" due to the interference of some conflict or train of thought. Freud (1901) used parapraxes (often but not always slips of the tongue or slips of the pen) to demonstrate the existence of unconscious mental processes in healthy individuals.

in language or reasoning stemmed from sources internal to the parent; that they occurred as a result of states of mental disorganization and conflict surrounding frightening experiences; and that they would eventually be found associated with the sporadic appearance of corresponding (frightened/frightening) *parental actions* which would in turn be predictive of infant disorganization (Main and Hesse, 1990). Above, we have reviewed a number of recent studies providing early corroboration for each of these hypotheses.

Here, we have introduced a coding system for identifying and scoring several kinds of parental behavior which we expect to find associated with an unresolved/disorganized mental state. In one subtype, the parent's alarm, and we propose that this may have particularly malignant consequences for the offspring. Overall, however, repeated exposure to interactions involving any of the FR subtypes described may increase the likelihood that the offspring of an unresolved/disorganized (traumatized) parent will develop a vulnerability to psychopathology.

In essence, we have advanced an extension of attachment theory which focuses upon a previously unrecognized aspect of the role of fear within the attachment relationship. Correspondingly, we have suggested a new mechanism by which the traumatic experiences of one individual can indirectly effect the development of a second. Finally, we have extended Bowlby's emphasis upon the role which direct experience plays in the development of psychopathology in the individual (Bowlby, 1969, 1980) by pointing to the powerful indirect influence of events which occurred in the previous generation and had become associated with anomalous fears, fantasies and ideation.

Thus, we have broadened the interpretation of what "real" events are to include the second-generation effects of unresolved trauma, and/or frightening ideation associated with experiences which would not necessarily have been considered inherently traumatic. From this point of view, the traumatic experience itself is of course not "real" for the second generation. What is real, however, is the developing child's interaction with a parent whose behavior at times reflects his or her original traumatic experiences, fears, and fantasies.

In sum, we have focused on the child's experiences as they are influenced by the traumatized and/or frightened parent, and have pointed to specific ways in which the second-generation effects of the parent's fears and experiences may create risk factors for psycho pathology. In keeping with a developmental pathways model (Sroufe and Rutter, 1984), we have suggested both (1) an immediate effect of interactions with a traumatized but not necessarily otherwise insensitive caregiver (disorganized infant attachment status), and correspondingly (2) an increased risk for the later development of psychological difficulties. The development of clinical levels of identifiable disorders will of course not normally depend solely on disorganized attachment with the primary caregiver in infancy, and will no doubt involve additional factors, including existing biological vulnerabilities. Here, for example, Walsh (1978) has reported that loss on the part of the parent within two years of the offspring's birth significantly increases the chances that a particular offspring within a given family will develop schizophrenia (Walsh, 1978; citing Orfanidis, p. 461). In other words, conditions which increase the likelihood that the parent was in an unresolved/disorganized state near the time of a particular birth have been found associated with the development of schizophrenia in biologically predisposed families (these and similar studies are reviewed in Hesse and van IJzendoorn, 1998, 1999). Other factors likely to increase the risk of unfavorable outcomes in later years include intervening trauma (Liotti, 1992; Ogawa et al., 1997), and disorganized attachment status with respect to the second parent.

REFERENCES

Abrams, K Y. (1999), Unpublished data. University of California at Berkeley.
———— and Rifkin, A. (1999), *Disorganized infant attachment and frightened/ frightening parental behavior: Evidence for new behaviors and new contexts (working title)*. Manuscript in preparation, University of California at Berkeley.
Ainsworth, M. D. S. (1967), *Infancy in Uganda: Infant care and the growth of love.* Baltimore: The Johns Hopkins Press.
———— (1969), Object relations, dependency and attachment: A theoretical review of the infant-mother relationship. *Child Development 40*, 969–1025.
———— (1991), Attachments and other affectional bonds. In P. Marris, J. Stevenson-Hinde, and C. Parkes (Eds.), *Attachment across the life cycle* (pp. 33–51). New York: Routledge.
———— Bell, S. M., and Stayton, D. J. (1971), Individual differences in Strange Situation behavior of one-year-olds. In H. R. Schaffer (Ed.), *The origins of human social relations* (pp. 17–57). London: Academic Press.
———— Blehar, M.C., Waters, E., and Wall, S. (1978), *Patterns of attachment: A psychological study of the Strange Situation*. Hillsdale, NJ: Erlbaum. Tavistock: London.
———— and Eichberg, C.G. (1991), Effects on infant-mother attachment of mother's unresolved loss of an attachment figure or other traumatic experience. In P. Marris,

J. Stevenson-Hinde, and C. Parkes (Eds.), *Attachment across the life cycle* (pp. 160–183). New York: Routledge.

Ammaniti, M., Speranza, A. M., and Candelori, C. (1996), Stability of attachment in children and intergenerational transmission of attachment. Stabilita dell'attacca-mento infantile e trasmissione intergenerazionale dell'attaccamento. *Psichiatria dell'Infancia e dell'Adolescenza, 63,* 313–332.

Benoit, D., and Parker, K. (1994), Stability and transmission of attachment across three generations. *Child Development 65,* 1444–1456.

Bowlby, J. (1944), Forty-four juvenile thieves: Their characters and home life. *International Journal of Psychoanalysis 25,* 107–127.

——— (1958), The nature of the child's tie to his mother. *International Journal of Psychoanalysis, 39,* 350–373.

——— (1980), *Attachment and loss: Vol. 3. Loss.* New York: Basic Books.

——— (1988), *A secure base: Parent-child attachment and healthy human development.* New York: Basic Books.

——— (1951), *Maternal care and mental health (WHO Monograph No. 2).* Geneva: World Health Organization.

——— (1969), *Attachment and loss: Vol. 1. Attachment.* New York: Basic Books.

——— (1973), *Attachment and loss: Vol 2. Separation.* New York: Basic Books.

——— (1982), *Attachment and loss: Vol. 1. Attachment* (2nd ed.). New York· Basic Books.

——— (1986), Videotaped autobiography given at the University of Virginia at Charlottesville. (M Main.).

Bretherton, I. (1992), The origins of attachment theory: John Bowlby and Mary Ainsworth. *Developmental Psychology 28,* 759–775.

Breuer, J., & Freud, S. (1960/1895), *Studies in Hysteria.* Boston: Beacon.

Buttner, A., Hieber, P., and Grossmann, K. (1997), *Unterschieden sich Mutter von desorganisierten und nicht desorganiserten Kindern in ihrem Verhalten in der Fremden Situation?* Poster bei der 13. Tagung Entwicklungaspsychologie, Wien, Sept.

Carlson, E. A.. (1998), A prospective longitudinal study of disorganized/disoriented attachment. *Child Development, 69,* 1970–1979.

Carlson, E. B., and Putnam, F. W. (1993), An update on the Dissociative Experiences Scale, *Dissociation, 7,* 16–27.

Carlson, V., Cicchetti, D., Barnett, D., and Braunwald, K. (1989), Disorganized/disoriented attachment relationships in maltreated infants. *Developmental Psychology 25,* 525–531.

Cassidy, J. (1999), The nature of the child's ties. In J. Cassidy and P. R. Shaver (Eds.), *Handbook of Attachment: Theory, research and clinical applications* (pp. 3–20). New York: The Guilford Press.

——— and Berlin, L. (1994), The insecure/resistant pattern of attachment: Theory and research. *Child Development 65,* 971–991.

Crittenden, P. M. (1985), Maltreated infants: Vulnerability and resilience. *Journal of Child Psychology & Psychiatry 26,* 85–96.

——— and Ainsworth, M. D. S. (1989), Child maltreatment and attachment theory. In D. Cicchetti and V. Carlson (Eds.), *Child maltreatment: Theory and research on the causes and consequences of child abuse and neglect* (pp. 432–463). New York: Cambridge University Press.

Darwin, C. (1872), *The expression of emotions in man and animals.* London: John Murray.

DeWolff, M. S., & van IJzendoorn, M. H. (1997), Sensitivity and attachment: A meta-analysis on parental antecedents of infant attachment. *Child Development 68*, 571–591.

Egeland, B., & Sroufe, L. A. (1981), Developmental sequelae of maltreatment in infancy. In R. Rizley and D. Cicchetti (Eds.), *Developmental Perspectives in Child Maltreatment* (pp. 77–92), San Francisco: Jossey-Bass.

Ellenberger, H. F. (1970), *The Discovery of the Unconscious: The History and Evolution of Dynamic Psychiatry*. New York: Basic Books.

Fonagy, P. (1999), Psychoanalytic theory from the viewpoint of attachment theory and research. In J. Cassidy and P. R. Shaver (Eds.), *Handbook of Attachment: Theory, research and clinical applications* (pp. 595–624). New York: The Guilford Press.

———— Steele, H. and Steele, M. (1991), Maternal representations of attachment during pregnancy predict the organization of infant-mother attachment at one year of age. *Child Development, 62*, 891–905.

Freud, S. (1920), *A General Introduction to Psychoanalysis*. New York: Boni and Liveright. (Authorized translation with a preface by G. Stanley Hall.)

———— (1901), *The Psychopathology of Everyday Life*. Standard Edition, Vol. 6, Hogarth Press, London, 1960.

George, C., & Solomon, J. (1996), Representational models of relationships: Links between caregiving and attachment. *Infant Mental Health, 17*, 198–216.

———— & ———— (1989), Internal working models of caregiving and security of attachment at age six. *Infant Mental Health, 10*, 222–237.

———— & ———— (1996), Representational models of relationships: Links between caregiving and attachment. *Infant Mental Health Journal, 17*, 198–216.

———— Kaplan, N., and Main, M. (1984, 1985, 1996), *Adult Attachment Interview*. Unpublished protocol, Department of Psychology, University of California, Berkeley.

Goldfarb, W. (1943), The effects of early institutional care on adolescent personality. *Journal of Experimental Education, 12*, 106–129.

———— (1945), Effects of psychological deprivation in infancy and subsequent stimulation. *American Journal of Psychiatry, 102*, 18–33.

Grossmann, K. E. (1997), *The development of attachment and psychological adaptation from the cradle to the grave*. Invited lecture, VIII European conference on Developmental Psychology, Rennes, France. September.

Hansburg, H. G. (1972), *Adolescent separation anxiety: A method for the study of adolescent separation problems*. Springfield, IL: Thomas.

Heinicke, C., and Westheimer, I. (1966), *Brief separations*. New York: International Universities Press.

Hertsgaard, L., Gunnar, M., Erickson, M. F. & Nachmias, M. (1995), Adrenocortical responses to the Strange Situation in infants with disorganized/disoriented attachment relationships. *Child Development, 66*, 1100–1106.

Hesse, E. (1999a), The Adult Attachment Interview: Historical and current perspectives. In J. Cassidy and P. R. Shaver (Eds.), *Handbook of Attachment: Theory, research and clinical applications* (pp. 395–433). New York: The Guilford Press.

———— (1996), Discourse, memory and the Adult Attachment Interview: A note with emphasis on the emerging Cannot Classify category. *Infant Mental Health Journal, 17*, 4–11.

———— (1999b), *Unclassifiable and Disorganized responses in the Adult Attachment Interview and in the Infant Strange Situation Procedure: Theoretical Proposals and Empirical Findings*. Unpublished doctoral dissertation, Leiden University.

———— and Main, M. (in press), Disorganization in infant and adult attachment: Descriptions, correlates and implications for developmental psychopathology. *Journal of the American Psychoanalytic Association.*

———— and van IJzendoorn, M. H. (in press), Propensities towards absorption are related to lapses in the monitoring of reasoning or discourse during the Adult Attachment Interview: A preliminary investigation. *Attachment and Human Development.*

Hesse, E., and van IJzendoorn, M. H. (1998), Parental loss of close family members and propensities towards absorption in offspring. *Developmental Science, 1,* 299–305.

Hilgard, E. R. (1977/1986), *Divided consciousness: Multiple controls in human thought and action.* New York: Wiley.

Hinde, R. A. (1966), *Animal behaviour: A synthesis of ethology and comparative psychology.* New York: McGraw-Hill.

———— (1974), *Biological bases of human social behavior.* New York: McGraw-Hill.

Hrdy, S. (1999), *Mother nature: A history of mothers, infants and natural selection.* New York: Pantheon.

Jacobsen, T., and Hofmann, V. (1997), Children's attachment representations: Longitudinal relations to school behavior and academic competency in middle childhood and adolescence. *Developmental Psychology, 33,* 703–710.

———— Edelstein, W. and Hofmann, V. (1994), A longitudinal study of the relation between representations of attachment in childhood and cognitive functioning in childhood and adolescence. *Developmental Psychology, 30,* 112–124.

———— Huss, M., Fendrich, M., Kruesi, M. P., and Ziegenhain, U. (1997), Children's ability to delay gratification: Longitudinal relations to mother-child attachment. *Journal of Genetic Psychology 158,* 411–426.

———— Ziegenhain, U., Muller, B., Rottmann, U., Hofmann, V. and Edelstein, W. (1992, September). *Predicting stability of mother-child attachment patterns in day-care children from infancy to age 6.* Poster presented at the Fifth World Congress of Infant Psychiatry and Allied Disciplines, Chicago.

Jacobvitz, D. (1998), *Frightening caregiving: Links with mother's loss and trauma.* Paper presented at the biennial meeting of the Southwestern Society for Research in Human Development. Galveston, Texas.

———— Hazen, N. L., and Riggs, S. (1997), *Disorganized mental processes in mothers, frightened/frightening behavior in caregivers, and disoriented, disorganized behavior in infancy.* Paper presented at the biennial meeting of the SRCD, Washington, D. C.

James, W. (1983), *The principles of psychology.* Cambridge: Harvard University Press. (Original work published in 1890).

Janet, P. (1965), *The major symptoms of hysteria.* New York: Hafner. (Original work published in 1907).

Kaplan, N. (1987), *Individual differences in six-year-old's thoughts about separation: Predicted from attachment to mother at age one.* Unpublished doctoral dissertation, University of California at Berkeley.

———— and Main, M. (1984, 1986), *Assessment of attachment organization through children's family drawings.* Unpublished manuscript, Department of Psychology, University of California at Berkeley.

Kermoian, R. and Campos, J. J. (1988), Locomotor experience: A facilitator of spatial cognitive development. *Child Development, 59,* 595–624.

Kihlstrom, J. F. (1997), Consciousness and me-ness. In J. D. Cohen and J. W. Schooler (Eds.), *Scientific approaches to consciousness* (pp. 451–468). Carnegie-Mellon symposium on cognition. New Jersey: Lawrence Erlbaum Associates, Inc.

Klagsbrun, M., and Bowlby, J. (1976), Responses to separation from parents: A clinical test for children. *British Journal of Projective Psychology, 21*, 7–21.

Klinnert, M. D., Campos, J. J., Sorce, J. F., Emde, R., and Svedja, M. (1983), Emotions as behavior regulators: Social referencing in infancy. In R. Plutchik and H. Kellerman (Eds.), *The emotions, Vol 2*. San Diego, CA: Academic Press.

Liotti, G. (1992), Disorganized/disoriented attachment in the etiology of the dissociative disorders. *Dissociation 5*, 196–204.

———— (1993), Disorganized attachment and dissociative experiences: An illustration of the developmental-ethological approach to cognitive therapy. In H. Rosen and K.T. Kuehlwein (Eds.), *Cognitive therapy in action* (pp. 213–239). San Francisco: Jossey-Bass.

———— (1999), Disorganization of attachment as a model for understanding dissociative psychopathology. In J. Solomon and C. George (Eds.), *Attachment disorganization* (pp. 291–317). New York: The Guilford Press.

Lyons-Ruth, K. (1996), Attachment relationships among children with aggressive behavior problems: The role of disorganized early attachment patterns. *Journal of Consulting and Clinical Psychology, 64*, 64–73.

———— and Jacobvitz, D. (1999), Attachment disorganization: Unresolved loss, relationship violence, and lapses in behavioral and attentional strategies. In J. Cassidy and P. R. Shaver (Eds.), *Handbook of Attachment: Theory, research and clinical applications* (pp. 520–554). New York: The Guilford Press.

———— Bronfman, E., and Parsons, E. (in press), Maternal disrupted affective communication, maternal frightened or frightening behavior, and disorganized infant attachment strategies. In J. Vondra and D. Barnett (Eds.), Atypical patterns of infant attachment: Theory, research and current directions. *Monographs of the Society for Research in Child Development*.

———— Repacholi, B., McLeod, S., and Silva, E. (1991), Disorganized attachment behavior in infancy: Short-term stability, maternal and infant correlates, and risk-related sub-types. *Development and Psychopathology, 3*, 377–396.

Main, M. (1973), *Exploration, play, and cognitive functioning as related to child-mother attachment*. Unpublished doctoral dissertation, The Johns Hopkins University.

———— (1979a), *Scale for disordered/disoriented infant behavior in response to the Main and Weston Clown Session*. Unpublished manuscript, University of California at Berkeley.

———— (1979b), The ultimate causation of some infant attachment phenomena: Further answers, further phenomena and further questions. *The Behavioral and Brain Sciences 2*, 640–643.

———— (1981), Avoidance in the service of attachment: A working paper. In K. Immelmann, G. Barlow, L. Petrinovitch, and M. Main (Eds.), *Behavioral development: The Blulefeld interdisciplinary project* (pp. 651–693). New York: Cambridge University Press.

———— (1990), Cross-cultural studies of attachment organization: Recent studies, changing methodologies and the concept of conditional strategies. *Human Development, 33*, 48–61.

———— (1995), Recent studies in attachment: Overview, with implications for clinical work. In S. Goldberg, R. Muir, and J. Kerr (Eds.), *Attachment Theory: Social, developmental and clinical perspectives*. Hillsdale, NJ: Analytic Press, Inc, pp. 407–474.

————— (1999), Epilogue. Attachment theory: Eighteen points with suggestions for future studies. In J. Cassidy and P. R. Shaver (Eds.), *Handbook of Attachment: Theory, Research and Clinical Applications* (pp. 845–888). New York: The Guilford Press.

————— (in press), The Adult Attachment Interview: Fear, attention, safety and discourse processes. *Journal of the American Psychoanalytic Association.*

————— and Stadtman, J. (1981), Infant response to rejection of physical contact by the mother: Aggression, avoidance and conflict. *Journal of the American Academy of Child Psychiatry, 20*: 2992–3007.

————— & Hesse, E. (1992–1998), Frightening, frightened, dissociated, deferential, sexualized and disorganized parental behavior: A coding system for frightening parent-infant interactions. Unpublished manuscript, University of California at Berkeley.

————— and Cassidy, J. (1988), Categories of response to reunion with the parent at age six: Predicted from infant attachment classifications and stable over a one-month period. *Developmental Psychology, 24*, 415–426.

————— and Goldwyn, R. (1984–1998), *Adult attachment scoring and classification system.* Unpublished manuscripts, Department of Psychology, University of California at Berkeley.

————— and Hesse, E. (1990), Parents' unresolved traumatic experiences are related to infant disorganized attachment status: Is frightened and/or frightening parental behavior the linking mechanism? In M. T. Greenberg, D. Cicchetti, and E. M. Cummings (Eds.), *Attachment in the preschool years: Theory, research, and intervention* (pp. 161–182). Chicago: University of Chicago Press.

————— and ————— (1992), Disorganized/disoriented infant behavior in the strange situation, lapses in the monitoring of reasoning and discourse during the parent's Adult Attachment Interview, and dissociative states. In M. Ammaniti and D. Stern (Eds.), *Attachment and psychoanalysis* (pp. 86-140). (Translated from the Italian).

————— and Morgan, H. (1996), Disorganization and disorientation in infant Strange Situation behavior: Phenotypic resemblance to dissociative states? In L. Michelson and W. Ray (Eds.), *Handbook of Dissociation: Theoretical, Empirical and Clinical Perspectives,* pp. 107–138. New York: Plenum.

————— and ————— (1986), Discovery of a new, insecure-disorganized/ disoriented attachment pattern. In T. B. Brazelton and M. W. Yogman (Eds.), *Affective development in infancy* (pp. 95–124). Norwood, NJ: Ablex.

————— and ————— (1990), Procedures for identifying infants as disorganized/ disoriented during the Ainsworth strange situation. In M. T. Greenberg, D. Cicchetti, and E. M. Cummings (Eds.), *Attachment in the preschool years: Theory, research, and intervention* (pp. 121–160). Chicago: University of Chicago Press.

————— and Weston, D. R. (1981), The quality of the toddler's relationship to mother and to father: Related to conflict behavior and the readiness to establish new relationships. *Child Development, 52*, 932–940.

————— Kaplan, N., and Cassidy, J. (1985), Security in infancy, childhood, and adulthood: A move to the level of representation. In I. Bretherton and E. Waters (Eds.), Growing points of attachment theory and research. *Monographs of the Society for Research in Child Development, 50* (Nos. 1–2, Serial No. 209), 66–104.

Manassis, K. Bradley, S., Goldberg, S., Hood, J., and Swinson, R. P. (1994), Attachment in mothers with anxiety disorders and their children. *J. American Academy of Child and Adolescent Psychiatry, 33*, 1106–1113.

Moss, E., Parent, S., Gosselin, C., Rousseau, D., and others (1996), Attachment and teacher-reported behavior problems during the preschool and early school-age period. *Development & Psychopathology, 8* :511–525.

───── Rousseau, D., Parent, S., St.-Laurent, D., and others (1998), Correlates of attachment at school age: Maternal reported stress, mother-child interaction, and behavior problems. *Child Development, 69*:1390–1405.

Ogawa, J. R., Sroufe, L. A., Weinfield, N. S., Carlson, E. A., and Egeland, B. (1997), Development and the fragmented self: Longitudinal study of dissociative symptomatology in a nonclinical sample. *Development and Psychopathology, 9*, 855–879.

Orvaschel, H., Puig-Antich, J., Chambers, W., Tabrizi, M. A., and Johnson, R. (1982), Retrospective assessment of prepubertal major depression with the Kiddie-SADS-E. *Journal of the American Academy of Child Psychiatry, 21*, 695–707.

Pederson, D. R., Gleason, K. E., Moran, G., and Bento, S. (1998), Maternal attachment representations, maternal sensitivity and the infant-mother attachment relationship. *Developmental Psychology, 34*, 925–933.

───── & Moran, G. (1996), Expressions of the attachment relationship outside of the Strange Situation. *Child Development 67*, 915–927.

Pipp-Siegel, S., Siegel, C. H., and Dean, J. (in press), Neurological aspects of the disorganized/disoriented attachment classification system: Differentiating quality of the attachment relationship from neurological impairment. In J. I. Vondra and D. Barnett (Eds.), Atypical attachment in infancy and early childhood among children at developmental risk. *Monographs of the Society for Research in Child Development*.

Prince, M. (1978), *The dissociation of a personality*. New York: Oxford University Press. (Original work published in 1905).

Putnam, F. W. (1985), Dissociation as a response to extreme trauma. In R. P. Kluft (Ed.), *The child antecedents of multiple personality*. Washington, D.C.: American Psychiatric Press.

Radke-Yarrow, M., Cummings, E. M., Kuczynski, L., and Chapman, M. (1985), Patterns of attachment in two- and three-year-olds in normal families with parental depression. Child Development, 56, 884–893.

Radojevic, M. (1992, July), *Predicting quality of infant attachment to father at 15 months from pre-natal paternal representations of attachment: An Australian contribution*. Paper presented at the XXV International Congress of Psychology, Brussels, Belgium, 19–25.

───── (1994), Mental representations of attachment among prospective Australian fathers. *Australian & New Zealand Journal of Psychiatry*, 28:505–511.

Robertson, J. and Robertson, J. (1971), Young children in brief separation: A fresh look. *Psychoanalytic study of the child, 26*, 264–315.

───── and Bowlby, J. (1952), Responses of young children to separation from their mothers. *Courrier Centre Internationale Enfance, 2*, 131–42.

Sandler, J. (1960), The background of safety. *International Journal of Psycho-analysis 41*, 352–365.

Schaffer, H. R. and Emerson, P. E. (1964), The development of social attachments in infancy. *Monographs of the Society for Research in Child Development* (Serial No. 94).

Schuengel, C., Van IJzendoorn, M. H. and Bakermans-Kranenburg, M. J. (1997), Attachment and loss: Frightening maternal behavior linking unresolved loss and disorganized infant attachment. In C. Schuengel, *Attachment, loss and maternal behavior: A study on intergenerational transmission* (pp. 40–58). Unpublished doctoral dissertation, Leiden University.

───── ───── ───── and Blom, M. (1997), *Frightening, frightened and/or dissociated behavior, unresolved loss and infant disorganization*. Paper presented at the biennial meeting of the Society for Research in Child Development, Washington, D. C.

───── ───── ───── (1999), Frightening maternal behavior linking unresolved loss and disorganized infant attachment. *Journal of Consulting and Clinical Psychology 67, 54–63.*

Siegel, D. (1999), *The developing mind: Towards a neurobiology of interpersonal experience.* New York: The Guilford Press.

Solomon, J. and George, C. (1999), The place of disorganization in attachment theory: Linking classic observations with contemporary findings. In J. Solomon and C. George (Eds.), *Attachment disorganization*, pp. 3–32. New York: The Guilford Press.

───── ───── & Ivins, B. (1987, April), *Mother-child interaction in the home and security of attachment at age six.* Paper presented at the biennial meeting of the Society for Research in Child Development, Baltimore.

───── ───── and DeJong, A. (1995), Children classified as controlling at age six: Evidence for disorganized representational strategies and aggression at home and at school. *Development and Psychopathology, 7,* 447–463.

Spangler, G. & Grossmann, K. E. (1993), Biobehavioral organization in securely and insecurely attached infant. *Child Development, 64,* 1439–1450.

Spiegel, D. (1990), Hypnosis, dissociation and trauma: Hidden and overt observers. In J. Singer (Ed.), *Repression and dissociation: Implications for personality theory, psychopathology, and health* (pp. 121–142), Chicago: University of Chicago Press.

Spitz, R. A. (1946), Anaclitic depression. *Psychoanalytic Study of the Child 2,* 313–342.

Sroufe, L. A. (1985), Attachment classification from the perspective of infant-caregiver relationships and infant temperament. *Child Development, 56,* 1–14.

───── & Waters, E. (1977), Heart-rate as a convergent measure in clinical and developmental research. *Merrill-Palmer Quarterly, 23,* 3–27.

───── and Rutter, M. (1984), The domain of developmental psychopathology. *Child Development, 55,* 1184–1199.

Steele, H., Steele, M. and Fonagy, P. (1996b), *Attachment in the sixth year of life.* Paper presented at the meetings of the International Congress of Psychology, Montreal.

───── ───── and ───── (1996a), Associations among attachment classifications of mothers, fathers and infants: Evidence for a relationship-specific perspective. *Child Development, 2,* 541–555.

Steele, M., Fonagy, P., Yabsley, S., Woolgar, M., and Croft, C. (1995, March), *Maternal representations of attachment during pregnancy predict the quality of children's doll play at five years of age.* Presented at the biennial meeting of the Society for Research in Child Development, Indianapolis, Indiana.

Strage, A., and Main, M. (1985), *Attachment and parent-child discourse patterns.* In M. Main (Chair), Attachment: A move to the level of representation. Paper presented at the biennial meeting of the Society for Research in Child Development, Toronto.

Tinbergen, N. (1951), *The study of instinct.* Oxford: Clarendon Press.

Troy, M., and Sroufe, L A. (1987), Victimization among pre-schoolers: The role of attachment-relationship theory. *Journal of the American Academy of Child and Adolescent Psychiatry 26,* 166–172.

True, M., Pasani, L., Ryan, R., and Oumar, F. (1998), *Maternal behaviors related to disorganized infant attachment in West Africa.* Paper presented at the annual meeting of the Western Psychological Association, Albuquerque, New Mexico.

van IJzendoorn, M. H. (1995), Adult attachment representations, parental responsiveness and infant attachment: A meta-analysis on the predictive validity of the Adult Attachment Interview. *Psychological Bulletin, 117*, 387–403.

———— and Kroonenberg, P. M. (1988), Cross-cultural patterns of attachment: A meta-analysis of the Strange Situation. *Child Development, 63*, 840–858.

———— Moran, G., Belsky, J., Pederson, D., Bakermans-Kranenburg, M., & Fisher, K. (in press), The similarity of siblings' attachments to their mother. *Child Development.*

———— and Bakermans-Kranenburg, M. (1996), Attachment representations in mothers, fathers, adolescents and clinical groups: A meta-analytic search for normative data. *Journal of Clinical and Consulting Psychology, 64*, 8–21.

———— and De Wolff, Marianne S. (1997), In search of the absent father—meta-analysis of infant-father attachment: A rejoinder to our discussants. *Child Development, 68*, 604–609.

———— Schuengel, C. and Bakermans-Kranenburg, M. J. (1999), Disorganized attachment in early childhood: Meta-analysis of precursors, concomitants and sequelae. *Development and Psychopathology*, in press.

Vaughn, B. E., and Bost, K. K. (1999), Attachment and temperament: Redundant, independent, or interacting influences on interpersonal adaptation and personality development? In J. Cassidy and P. R. Shaver (Eds.), *Handbook of Attachment: Theory, Research and Clinical Applications* (pp. 198–225). New York: The Guilford Press.

Volkmar, F. R., and Siegel, A. E. (1979), Young children's responses to discrepant social communications. *Journal of Child Psychology and Psychiatry, 20*, 139–149.

———— Hoder, E. L., and Siegel, A. E. (1980), Discrepant social communications. *Developmental Psychology 16*, 495–505.

Walsh, F. W. (1978), Concurrent grandparent death and birth of schizophrenic offspring: An intriguing finding. *Family Process, 17*, 457–463.

Ward, M. J., and Carlson, E.A. (1995), The predictive validity of the adult attachment interview for adolescent mothers. *Child Development, 66*, 69–79.

Wartner, U. G., Grossmann, K., Fremmer-Bombik, E., and Suess, G. (1994), Attachment patterns at age six in South Germany: Predictability from infancy and implications for preschool behavior. *Child Development, 65*, 1014–1027.

Weinfield, S., Sroufe, L. A., Egeland, B. and Carlson, E. A. (1999), The nature of individual differences in infant-caregiver attachment. In J. Cassidy and P. R. Shaver (Eds.), *Handbook of Attachment: Theory, Research and Clinical Applications* (pp. 68–88). New York: The Guilford Press.

Winnicott, D. W. (1974), Fear of breakdown. *International Review of Psychoanalysis, 1*, 103–107.

Department of Psychology
University of California at Berkeley
Berkeley, CA 94720
(fax) 510-642-5293

Attachment Theory and Psychoanalysis: Further Differentiation Within Insecure Attachment Patterns

KENNETH N. LEVY, Ph.D.
SIDNEY J. BLATT, Ph.D.

THEORETICAL EMPHASES IN PSYCHOANALYSIS HAVE CHANGED over the years from classical drive theory to an increasing focus on the role of object relationships and object representation in personality development and psychopathology (e.g., Winnicott, 1960; Blatt, 1974; Mahler, Pine, and Bergman, 1975; Kernberg, 1976; Blatt & Lerner, 1983a). Central to object relational models is the concept of mental representation of self and other. Mental representations are enduring cognitive-affective psychological structures that provide templates for processing and organizing information so that new experiences are assimilated to existing mental structures. These mental schemas guide an individual's behavior, particularly in interpersonal relationships (Blatt & Lerner, 1983b). These cognitive–affective schemas or mental representations of self and other develop over the life cycle. They have conscious and unconscious cognitive, affective, and experiential components that derive from significant early interpersonal experiences. These cognitive–affective schemas can involve veridical representations of consensual reality, idiosyncratic and unique constructions, or primitive and pathological distortions that suggest

Kenneth Levy is a graduate student in the Clinical Psychology Doctoral Program at the City University of New York and a psychology intern at The New York Presbyterian Hospital, Weill School of Medicine, Cornell Medical Center.

Sidney J. Blatt is a member of the Departments of Psychiatry and Psychology, Yale University, New Haven, CT.

psychopathology (Blatt, 1991, 1995). They also reflect the individual's developmental level and such important aspects of psychic life as impulses, affects, drives, and fantasies (Sandler and Rosenblatt, 1962; Beres and Joseph, 1970; Blatt, 1974).

This shift to object relations theories within psychoanalysis is consistent with and, in part, influenced by research in infant development (e.g., Emde, 1983; Litchenberg, 1985; Stern, 1985) and by attachment theory and research (e.g., Bowlby, 1973, 1980, 1982; Ainsworth et al., 1978; Sroufe, 1983; Main, Kaplan, and Cassidy, 1985; Main and Cassidy, 1988). Despite its historical links with psychoanalytic and object relations perspectives, attachment theory has been adopted primarily by investigators in developmental psychology concerned about "normal" development and, until recently, has been relatively neglected by psychoanalytic clinicians. The recent theoretical and empirical work of Mary Main and her colleagues (Main and Goldwyn, 1985; Main et al., 1985; Main and Cassidy, 1988; Main and Hesse, 1990), elaborating on the nature of internal working models of attachment, provides further opportunity to integrate attachment theory and research with object relational theories of mental representations in psychoanalysis.

Mental representations in object relations theory are generally analogous to the internal working models discussed in attachment theory. Both attachment theory (e.g., Ainsworth, 1969; Bowlby, 1980; Bretherton, 1985) and object relations theory (e.g., Fairbairn, 1952; Winnicott, 1960; Jacobson, 1964; Blatt, 1974; Kernberg, 1976) postulate that "mental representations," or "internal working models" of self and others, emerge from early relationships with caregivers and then act as heuristic guides for subsequent interpersonal relationships influencing expectations, feelings, and general patterns of behavior (Slade and Aber, 1992; Diamond and Blatt, 1994). Despite their convergences, psychoanalytic concepts of mental representations and concepts of internal working models in attachment theory are different in important respects. Mental representations and internal working models are not just different terms that describe the same phenomena. Compared with internal working models of attachment theory, the concept of representations in object relations theory has a more epigenetic developmental quality (Blatt, 1974; Diamond and Blatt, 1994; Levy, Blatt, and Shaver, 1998). Mental representations in psychoanalytic theory proceed through a developmental sequence, becoming increasingly complex, abstract, symbolic, and verbally mediated (Freud, 1914; Blatt, 1974, 1995; Horowitz, 1977).

This paper examines some of the ways in which object relations and attachment theories can inform each other and thus provide a broad-ranging theoretical model of personality development and psycho-pathology across a wider developmental spectrum. Recent attachment research provides a valuable heuristic framework for conducting psychoanalytic research, enriching psychoanalytic clinicians and investigators. And psychoanalytic concepts can inform and facilitate theory and research in developmental psychology and attachment theory to place their findings in a broad theoretical context. With this in mind we review the current status of the attachment literature with children and adults from both a developmental and social psychologi-cal perspective. The primary purpose of this paper is to address the importance of distinguishing among different developmental levels of mental representations and how these differences can enrich and extend our understanding of various attachment patterns.

Attachment Theory

Bowlby, a British psychiatrist, was trained as a physician and psycho-analyst early in this century when object relations approaches to psychoanalysis were first beginning to be formulated (see Karen, 1994, for an account of Bowlby's intellectual development). Bowlby was trained in the period when Anna Freud, Melanie Klein, and Donald Winnicott and others were beginning to apply psychoanalytic concepts to the study and treatment of children, during the period of transition in psychoanalysis from a one-person, closed system psychology primarily concerned with drive forces and discharge thresholds to two-person, more open systems, object relational theo-ries. Bowlby clashed with his supervisor Melanie Klein over the issue of whether to involve the mother in the psychoanalytic treatment of a child. This difference in focus was the beginning of Bowlby's eventual estrangement from the psychoanalytic community. In contrast to object relations theorists such as Winnicott who retained much of Freud's emphasis on sexual and aggressive drives and fantasies, Bowlby's attachment theory focused on the affective bond in close interpersonal relationships. Bowlby believed that Klein and other psychoanalysts overestimated the role of infantile fantasy, neglecting the role of actual experiences. Moreover, Bowlby boldly proposed that internal working models "are tolerably accurate reflections of the experiences those individuals have actually had" (Bowlby, 1973, p. 235). In contrast to Bowlby, Fairbairn (1952), Guntrip (1971), and Winnicott (1965) retained enough ties to drive theory in terms of unconscious fantasy and infantile distortion that they avoided the banishment that Bowlby experienced. Additionally, in contrast to most psychoanalysts of the time, Bowlby was also empirically minded. Rather than draw inferences about childhood from the free associations, dreams, transferences, and other mental productions of adults primarily seen in psychoanalytic treatment, Bowlby wanted to study and work directly with children. His focus was on the observable behavior of infants and their interactions with their caregivers, especially their mothers, and he encouraged prospective studies of the effects of early attachment relationships on personality development. In this sense he was again different than many of his object relations colleagues who focused instead on adults' mental representations of self and others in close relationships, often revealed during psychoanalysis and psychotherapy, although these colleagues also believed that these representations were the result of early relationships with parents.

While Bowlby was critical of certain aspects of classic psychoanalytic formulations, his work clearly falls within the framework of psychoanalysis because he retained and extended many of Freud's clinical and developmental insights. Central to Bowlby, as with Freud, is the view that notable early experiences have significant impact on subsequent development. Attachment theory emerged from Bowlby's observations in England during World War II of the pervasive disruptive consequences of deprivation of contact with the mother in children temporarily separated from their primary caregiver (usually the mother) because of the war; he observed that "the young child's hunger for his mother's love and presence is as great as his hunger for food" and that her absence inevitably generates "a powerful sense of loss and anger" (Bowlby, 1969, p. xiii). Bowlby identified a clear and predictable sequence of three emotional reactions that typically occur subsequent to the separation of an infant from its primary caregiver:

first, protest that involves crying, active searching, and resistance to others' soothing efforts; then despair, which is a state of passivity and obvious sadness; and then detachment, which involves an active, seemingly defensive disregard for and avoidance of the mother if she returns. Successive, systematic observation revealed that the typical infant checks back regularly, visually and/or physically, to ensure the mother is available and responsive. If the mother moves or directs her attention elsewhere, the child attempts to recapture that attention through eye contact, smiling, vocalizing (babbling, crying), or returning to her side (including clinging and following). When the attachment system is strongly activated, most children cry and seek physical contact with their primary caregiver. When the attachment system is idle, children play happily, smile easily, share toys and discoveries with their caregiver, and display warm interest in others. The attachment system is especially prone to activation under conditions of anxiety, fear, illness, and fatigue. These observations were further elaborated by Bowlby's (1944) classic study of forty-four delinquent children.

Based on ethological theory, Bowlby postulated that the caregiver–infant attachment bond is a complex, instinctually guided behavioral system that has functioned throughout human evolution to protect the infant from danger and predators. Secure attachment to the mother in infancy derives primarily from the mother's reliable and sensitive provision of security and love as well as food and warmth. Consistent differences occur, however, in the degree to which infant–mother relationships are characterized by experiences of security. Some mothers are slow or erratic in responding to their infant's cries; other mothers regularly intrude into or interfere with their infant's desired activities (sometimes to force "affection" on the infant at a particular moment). The infants of these mothers cry more often and explore less (even in the mother's presence) than securely attached infants, and they often mingle active seeking of the mother with overt expressions of anger and seem generally anxious. In addition, some infants may eventually try to avoid mothers who previously had frequently rebuffed or rejected their infant's attempts to establish physical contact with her. These distinctions led investigators (e.g., Ainsworth) to contrast secure attachment with two types of insecure attachment that they called avoidant and anxious ambivalent.

Bowlby (1973) and Ainsworth (1969) formulated that infants construct mental representations or affective–cognitive schemas of the self and of others, as well as develop expectations about interpersonal relations based on transactions with their attachment figures. These "internal working mental models" (Ainsworth, 1969; Bowlby, 1973), or mental representations, are the building blocks of personality development, and they direct and shape future interpersonal relationships. The continuity of these mental models over time is rooted in the nature of concepts of self and others, as well as interpersonal expectations constructed by the child. This internal working model of the interaction between self and others guides subsequent interpersonal relationships. For example, an infant whose needs are typically left unmet may develop a model of others as unreliable and uncaring and of the self as unlovable. Consequently, the neglected infant and child may, as an adult, believe that each new person will prove to be inaccessible, uncaring, and unresponsive. Conversely, the child whose needs have been addressed in a consistent loving and supportive manner may subsequently regard others as dependable and trustworthy and the self as lovable and attractive.

Based on Bowlby's attachment theory, Ainsworth conducted a seminal study to observe the effects of childbearing techniques employed by mothers on the development of a child's attachment patterns. Ainsworth and her colleagues (Ainsworth et al., 1978) developed a technique called the "strange situation," which involves eight standard episodes staged in a playroom through which the infant, the caregiver, and a "stranger" interact in a comfortable setting and the behaviors of the infant are observed. First, the baby has the chance to explore toys while the mother is present. Gradually, a stranger enters, converses with the mother, and invites the baby to play. Then the mother leaves the baby with the stranger, returns for a reunion, and then the baby is left alone; the stranger then returns, and finally, the mother returns for a second reunion. Ainsworth was able to categorize infants with considerable reliability into three distinct groups based on their reunion behavior with their mothers after this brief separation. Based on observations of infants and their caretakers, Ainsworth et al. (1978) identified three distinct patterns or styles of infant–mother attachment: secure (63% of the dyads tested), avoidant (21%), and anxious–ambivalent (16%). All three types of infants are *attached* to their mothers, yet significant individual differences in the quality of that attachment relationship can be identified and measured reliably. The *avoidant* dyad is characterized by a quiet distance in the mother's presence, acting unaware of the mother's departure, and avoiding the mother upon reunion. The *anxious–ambivalent* dyad is characterized by much emotional protest and anger on the part of the infant. The baby acts extremely distressed on the mother's departure and becomes angry and resistant. The baby approaches the mother for attention but angrily resists being picked up, yet is clingy, dependent, often crying, and unable to be soothed and comforted upon the mother's return. The *secure* dyad is characterized by the child's confident use of the mother as a "secure base" (Bowlby, 1988) to explore the playroom with great ease and comfort in the mother's presence. This exploration diminishes upon the mother's departure, but the child greets the mother on her return with great enthusiasm and seeks proximity and interaction with the mother, resumes exploration of the environment, and is able to play again independently. These findings (Ainsworth et al., 1978) have been replicated and extended by many subsequent investigators in a number of different cultures (e.g., Waters, Wippman, and Sroufe, 1979; Erikson, Sroufe, and Egeland, 1985; Main et al., 1985; Sroufe and Fleeson, 1986; see reviews by Bretherton, 1985 and Paterson and Moran, 1988).

Consistent with Bowlby's theory, these three attachment styles are closely associated with differences in caretaker warmth and responsiveness (Ainsworth et al., 1971, 1974, 1978; Blehar, Lieberman, & Ainsworth, 1977, Maslin and Bates, 1983; Belsky, Rovine, and Taylor, 1984; Egeland and Farber, 1984; Grossmann et al., 1985; Main et al., 1985; Goldberg et al., 1986; Smith and Pederson, 1988; Crowell and Feldman, 1988; Pederson et al., 1990; Isabella and Belsky, 1991; see van IJzendoorn, 1995, for metaanalysis). Ainsworth and colleagues (1971, 1975) and Grossmann et al. (1985), in a German sample, found that maternal sensitivity during infancy was strongly predictive of the security of infants' attachment to their mothers. Other studies have also provided strong support for the link between mother's sensitivity and attachment security of her infant. For example, mothers of securely attached, in contrast to mothers of insecurely attached, infants tend to hold their babies more carefully, tenderly, and for longer periods of time during early infancy (Main et al., 1985).

Additionally, mothers of securely attached infants respond more frequently to their infants' crying, show more affection when holding the baby, are more likely to acknowledge the baby with a smile or conversation when entering the baby's room, and are better at feeding the baby because of their attention to the baby's signals compared to mothers of babies later independently judged to be insecurely attached. These findings are consistent with findings from studies of maternal sensitivity (e.g., Crowell and Feldman, 1988) in which the mother's level of sensitivity to her infant's communication significantly predicted the infant's attachment style (Smith and Pedersen, 1988).

A number of longitudinal studies have investigated the influence of infant attachment styles on subsequent functioning and adaptive potential. Securely attached infants as preschoolers are cooperative, popular with peers, and highly resilient and resourceful (Sroufe, 1983) and at age 6 are relaxed and friendly and converse with their parents in a free-flowing and easy manner (Main and Cassidy, 1988). Insecure avoidant infants as preschoolers appear emotionally insulated, hostile, and antisocial (Sroufe, 1983) and later tend to distance themselves from their parents' and ignore their parents initiatives in conversation (Main and Cassidy, 1988). Anxious–resistant or preoccupied insecure infants are tense and impulsive as toddlers and passive and helpless in preschool (Sroufe, 1983) and later show a mixture of insecurity and hostile behavior in interaction with their parents (Main and Cassidy, 1988).

Two studies (Grossman and Grossman, 1991; Elicker, Englund, and Sroufe, 1993) followed children for as long as 10 years after their assessment in the strange situation and found central personality variables and social behavior predictable over that decade. Elicker, Englund, and Sroufe (1993) report that infant attachment style, even after controlling for the infant's adjustment and home environment, reliably predicted the child's social skill and self-confidence 10 years later. Specifically, secure attachment in infancy predicted more positive relationships with teachers and more socially adept, close friendships with peers at age 11. Waters et al. (1995) followed 50 individuals for 20 years and found a 64% stability in attachment classification (actually greater than 70% stability for individuals with no major negative life events and less than 50% stability for those who lost a parent, endured parental divorce, etc.). Thus longitudinal research, though still preliminary, suggests that attachment patterns identified during infancy are stable over time (Bretherton, 1985), even into early adulthood (age 20). Although the available evidence indicates that attachment classifications are fairly stable over extended periods of time, various factors contribute to their relative stability and change, including temperament, continuing relationships with the same family members, negative life events, change-resistant internal working models, and behavior patterns that produce self-fulfilling prophecies. All of these factors most likely play a significant role (see Rothbard and Shaver, 1994, for a review of research on continuity), but further research is needed to elaborate how and to what degree these various factors contribute to the stability or change of attachment styles.

Adult Attachment

Based on Bowlby's (1977) contention that the attachment system is active "from the cradle to the grave," various investigators (e.g., Main et al., 1985; Hazan and Shaver, 1987, 1990; West and Sheldon, 1988; Sperling, 1988; Sperling and Berman, 1991) independently began to apply the concepts of attachment theory to the study of adult behavior and personality.

Based on Ainsworth's differentiation of types of patterns of attachment, Main et al. (1985) developed an interview to assess adults' internal working models—the security of the adult's overall model of attachment and of the self in attachment experiences—in order to study the relationship of behaviors in adults to the quality of the attachment to their parents. The interview inquires into "descriptions of early relationships and attachment related events for the adult's sense of the way these relationships and events had affected adult personality; by probing for both specific corroborative and contradictory memories of parents and the relationship with parents" (Main et al., 1985, p. 98). Three major patterns of adult attachment were initially identified: secure, detached, and enmeshed; two additional styles were subsequently identified: the disorganized style and the unclassifiable style. The first three categories parallel the attachment classifications originally identified in studies of children (Ainsworth et al., 1978), and the disorganized style parallels a pattern later described in infants (Main and Solomon, 1990).

Attachment from a Social Psychological Perspective

In contrast to Main's focus on the study of the relationship of adults with their parents, Hazan and Shaver (1987; Shaver, Hazan, and Bradshaw, 1988), from a social psychological perspective, applied the childhood attachment paradigm to the study of adult romantic love. Hazan and Shaver (1987) developed questionnaires to assess attachment styles in adult relationships. They reasoned that the same three attachment styles identified in children might exist in adolescence and adulthood and have important implications for the formation of romantic relationships (Shaver and Hazan, 1987; Shaver et al., 1988). They translated Ainsworth's descriptions of the three infant attachment types into a single-item measure appropriate to adult romantic relationships. Following Ainsworth et al. (1978), they labeled the three types of adult attachments as secure, avoidant, and anxious–ambivalent. Subjects were first asked to characterize themselves as secure, avoidant, or anxious–ambivalent in romantic relationships based on three descriptions; they were then asked to respond to questions related to their "most important" experiences of romantic love, their mental models of self and relationships, and their memories of childhood relationships with parents (attachment history). Hazan and Shaver (1987) found approximately the same proportions of the three attachment types in adolescents and young adults (secure—62%, avoidant—23%, and anxious–ambivalent—15%) that Ainsworth et al. (1978) had obtained in the studies of infants. Similar percentages have been found in subsequent studies using Hazan and Shaver's measure in at least three different industrialized countries (Collins and Read, 1990; Feeney and Nollar, 1990; Muklincer, Florian, and Tolmacz, 1990).

Hazan and Shaver (1987) also found significant links between self-reported romantic attachment style and the quality of interpersonal relationships. Secure subjects' experiences of love were characterized by caring, intimacy, supportiveness, and understanding; avoidant subjects by fear of intimacy; and anxious ambivalent subjects by emotional instability, obsession, physical attraction, and the desire for union. Additionally, greater loneliness was found among insecure subjects. In a subsequent study, Hazan and Shaver (1990) also reported that secure subjects, in contrast to both groups of insecure subjects, reported less depression, anxiety, hostility, and physical illness than insecure subjects. Avoidant subjects tended to be satisfied with work but not with their coworkers and, instead, preferred to work alone. Anxious ambivalent subjects, in contrast, preferred to work with others and did not enjoy the actual work but more the people with whom they worked.

An important recent development in attachment research has been the contributions of (Bartholomew, 1990; Bartholomew and Horowitz, 1991) who noticed an inconsistency between conception of avoidance in formulations of Main and those of Hazen and Shaver. Bartholomew noted that Main's prototype of the adult avoidant style (assessed in the context of parenting) is more defensive, denial-oriented, and overtly unemotional than Hazan and Shaver's avoidant attachment prototype (assessed in the context of romantic attachment), which seems more vulnerable, conscious of emotional pain, and "fearful." Thus, Bartholomew viewed Main's avoidant style as predominantly dismissing, whereas Hazan and Shaver's avoidant style seemed predominantly fearful.

Consistent with Bowlby, Bartholomew conceptualized adult attachment styles in terms of the combination of the representational models of self and others that purportedly underlie these styles. It became evident to Bartholomew that the four attachment categories (Figure 1) could be arrayed in a two-dimensional space, with one dimension being the "model of self" (positive versus negative) and the other being the "model of others" (positive versus negative).

For secure individuals, models of self and other are both generally positive. For preoccupied or anxious-ambivalent individuals, the model of others is positive (i.e., relationships are attractive), but the model of self is not. For dismissing individuals, the reverse is true: the somewhat defensively maintained model of self is positive, whereas the model of others is negative (i.e., intimacy in relationships is regarded with caution or avoided). Fearful individuals have relatively negative models of both self and others.

To assess both types of avoidant styles, dismissing and fearful, Bartholomew developed a four-category interview that parallels

Figure 1 Bartholomew's Analysis of Four Adult Attachment Styles in Terms of Two Dimensions, Model of Self and Model of Other.

	Model of Self	
	Positive	Negative
	SECURE	**PREOCCUPIED**
	Comfortable with	Preoccupied with
Positive	intimacy and	relationships
	autonomy	
Model of Other		
	DISMISSING	**FEARFUL**
	Dismissing of	Fearful of intimacy;
Negative	intimacy;	Socially avoidant
	Counterdependent	

Main's Adult Attachment Interview (AAI) and a four-category self-report measure that parallels the work of Hazan and Shaver. In a number of studies, Bartholomew found that the personality styles of the two avoidant types were quite distinct. Fearful avoidant individuals are characterized as low in self-esteem, hesitant, shy, lonely, vulnerable, dependent, self-critical, afraid of rejection, and lacking in social confidence. On the other hand, dismissingly avoidant individuals are characterized as high in self-esteem, socially self-confident, unemotional, defensive, independent, cynical, critical of others, distant from others, and more interested in achievement than in relationships. Although dismissing avoidant individuals rated themselves as high in self-esteem, their peers saw them as hostile and socially autocratic. This finding is consistent with Kobak and Sceery (1988) who, using the AAI, found that avoidant subjects rated themselves as socially adept and psychologically sound, whereas their peers viewed them as more hostile and less ego-resilient. Thus, fearfully avoidant individuals are characterized by a conscious desire for relatedness which is inhibited by fears of its consequences, whereas dismissing avoidant subjects are characterized by a defensive denial of the need and/or desire for relatedness. Research is accumulating that supports the importance of Bartholomew's distinction between fearful and dismissing types of avoidant attachment (see Brennan, Shaver, and Tobey, 1990; Bartholomew and Horowitz, 1991; Horowitz, Rosenberg, and Bartholemew, 1993; Feeney, Nollar, and Hanrahan, 1994; Levy, Blatt, and Shaver, 1998).

Although the AAI category system, Hazan and Shaver's three-category typology, Bartholomew's four-category typology, and several variations of these conceptual frameworks are all rooted in Bowlby and Ainsworth's theory and research, they are not conceptually identical (e.g., some are more clearly dimensional than others, and some focus on parenting whereas others focus on romantic relationships), and they have generated different kinds of measures. The AAI is scored primarily in terms of indicators of "current state of mind," such as awkward pauses, gaps in memory, incoherent discourse, and other signs of defensiveness. The self-report measures, such as Bartholomew's and Hazan and Shaver's, tap self-characterizations of beliefs, feelings, and behaviors in romantic or other close relationships. Comparisons between the AAI and self-report categories have typically failed to correspond (Borman and Cole, 1993; Crowell, Treboux, and Waters, 1993; Shaver, Belsky, and Brennan, in press). Studies that have related the dimensional coding scales from the AAI to the self-report measures, however, have found that they are significantly related, even if the two categorical typologies were not significantly related (Shaver, Belsky, and Brennan, in press). Additionally, while it is true that there was no criterion such as children's performance in the Strange Situation used in the development of the Hazan and Shaver or Bartholomew measures, there is considerable construct validity in the realms of personality and adult relationships for these measures. In sum, a host of studies since 1987 like Hazan and Shaver's brief measure and various extensions of it have been sufficiently precise (see Scharfe and Bartholomew, 1994) to generate a large and coherent body of evidence supporting their construct validity. Adult attachment styles have significantly predicted relationship outcomes (e.g., satisfaction, breakups, commitment), patterns of coping with stress, couple communication, and even phenomena such as religious experiences and patterns of career development as well as studies that make behavioral predictions (Bartholomew and Horowitz, 1991; Hazan and Hutt, 1991; Mikulincer and Nachshon, 1991; Simpson, Rholes, and Nelligan, 1992; Feeney and Kirpatrick, 1995; Fraley and Shaver, 1998; for reviews see Shaver and Hazan, 1993; Hazan and Shaver, 1994; Shaver and Clark). Moreover, Rholes, Simpson, and Blakely (1995) used self-report measures to assess attachment in a study of the quality of mother-child relationships.

Similar to studies relating the AAI derived attachment styles to outcomes in the child strange situation, they found that avoidant mothers did not feel as close to their preschool children as did more secure mothers, and they behaved in less supportive ways toward their children during a laboratory teaching task. Still there are no studies relating the self-report measures to children's attachment patterns derived from the Strange Situation. Taken together; however, findings using self-report measures are highly consistent with those using the interview method, even if the two categorical typologies are not significantly related (Crowell, Fraley, and Shaver, 1999).

Bartholomew and Shaver (1998) contend that recent examination of several studies based on Bartholomew's measures and either the AAI or Hazan and Shaver's measure suggests a rough continuum ranging from the AAI (an interview measure focused on parenting issues and coded categorically rather than dimensionally), through Bartholomew's parental attachment and peer/romantic interviews and self-report measure, to Shaver and Hazan's self-report measure. Methods that lie close to each other on this continuum are more highly related empirically, but factor analyses or structural equation models based on several measures consistently indicate the presence of an underlying latent construct (see Griffin and Bartholomew, 1994a, b), which Bartholomew and Shaver (1998) interpret as reflecting a common core that is established in childhood. These attachment orientations may become differentiated with development and social experience. Several other investigators have replicated and extended the findings of Hazan and Shaver and Bartholomew (Levy and Davis, 1988; Collins and Read, 1990; Feeney and Noller, 1990; Mikulincer et al., 1990; Simpson, 1990; Simpson, Rholes, and Nelligan, 1992), demonstrating that these measures of attachment style in adults are precise (see Scharfe and Bartholomew, 1994) and generated a large and coherent body of evidence supporting their construct validity (for reviews see Shaver and Hazan, 1993; Hazan and Shaver, 1994; Shaver and Clark, 1994).

Adult attachment styles have significantly predicted relationship outcomes (e.g., satisfaction, breakups, commitment), patterns of coping with stress, couple communication, and even phenomena such as religious experiences and patterns of career development, as well as behavioral predictions (Brennan and Shaver, 1994; Feeney and

Kirkpatrick, 1996; Hazan and Hutt, 1991; Kirkpartrick and Davis, 1994; Mikulincer and Nachshon, 1991; Simpson et al., 1992). Thus, the findings of these studies do not seem to be a function of some kind of a pervasive self-report response bias or set.

Developmental Levels of Representation and Attachment

While attachment theory is a developmental theory, attachment theorists and researchers, have, ironically, neglected to integrate a developmental perspective into this work, particularly when considering the concept of internal working models. Attachment styles are described as essentially static, and thus, the concept of attachment styles could be enriched considerably by the introduction of a developmental dynamic. Compared with attachment theory's somewhat fixed notion of "internal working models," the concept of "representations" in object relations theory has a more epigenetic, developmental quality (Blatt, 1974; Diamond and Blatt, 1994; Levy, Blatt, and Shaver, 1998). Psychoanalytic theorists (Blatt, 1974, 1995; Freud, 1914; Horowitz, 1977) view modes of representation as proceeding through a developmental sequence, becoming increasingly complex, abstract, symbolic, and verbally mediated. Thus, psychoanalysis can contribute to the study of attachment through the identification of developmental levels of representation.

Blatt and his colleagues (Blatt, 1974, 1995; Blatt and Lerner, 1983), integrating psychoanalytic theory and the cognitive developmental perspective of Piaget (1952) and Werner (1948), suggest that the cognitive and affective components of representations of self and other develop epigenetically—becoming increasingly accurate, articulated, and conceptually complex. According to this approach, higher levels of representation evolve from and extend lower levels; thus, new representational modes are increasingly more comprehensive and effective than earlier modes of representation. Following these epigenetic principles, Blatt and colleagues stress that representations of self and others can range from global, diffuse, fragmentary, and inflexible to increasingly differentiated, flexible, and hierarchically organized.

These formulations are consistent with Kernberg's (1976) view that representations derive from relationships to primary caregivers interpersonal experiences are stored in memory (internalized) and that

Table 1 Differentiation-Relatedness of Self and Object Representations.

Level/Scale Point	Description
1. Self/other boundary compromise	Basic sense of physical cohesion or integrity of representations are lacking or are breached.
2. Self/other boundary confusion	Self and other are represented as physically intact and separate, but feelings and thoughts are amorphous, undifferentiated, or confused. Description may consist of a single global impressionistic quality or a flood of details with a sense of confusion and vagueness.
3. Self/other mirroring	Characteristics of self and other, such as physical appearance or body qualities, shape, or size, are virtually identical.
4. Self/other idealization or denigration	Attempt to consolidate representations based on unitary, unmodulated idealization, or denigration. Extreme, exaggerated, one-sided descriptions.
5. Semi-differentiated, tenuous consolidation of representations through splitting (polarization) and/or by an emphasis on concrete part properties	Marked oscillation between dramatically opposite qualities or an emphasis on manifest external features.
6. Emergent, ambivalent constancy (cohesion) of self and an emergent sense of relatedness	Emerging consolidation of disparate aspects of self and other in a somewhat hesitant, equivocal, or ambivalent integration. A list of appropriate conventional characteristics, but they lack a sense of uniqueness. Tentative movement toward a more individuated and cohesive sense of self and other.
7. Consolidated constant (stable) self and other in unilateral relationships	Thoughts, feelings, needs, and fantasies are differentiated and modulated. Increasing tolerance for and integration of disparate aspects. Distinguishing qualities and characteristics. Sympathetic understanding of others.
8. Cohesive, individuated, empathically related self and others	Cohesive, nuanced, and related sense of self and others. A definite sense of identity and an interest in interpersonal relationships and a capacity to understand the perspective of others.
9. Reciprocally related integrated unfolding self and others	Cohesive sense of self and others in reciprocal relationships that transform both the self and the other in complex, continually unfolding ways.
10. Creative, integrated constructions of self and other in empathic, reciprocally attuned relationships	Integrated reciprocal relations with an appreciation that one contributes to the construction of meaning in complex interpersonal relationships.

through the process of internalization. Kernberg proposes that early these memories consist of three parts: (a) representation of self, (b) a representation of others, and (c) the affective tone characteristic of these representations. For Kernberg, the degree of differentiation and integration of these representations of self and other, along with their affective valance, defines important aspects of the individual's personality structure. Development proceeds as representations of self and others become increasingly differentiated and integrated. More mature representations allow for the integration of positive and negative elements and for the tolerance of ambivalence and contradiction in feelings about self and others. More integrated and mature representations have greater richness and complexity.

Because internal working models of attachment research are limited to several prototypic attachment transactions, they lack the potential intricacy, complexity, and detail of psychoanalytic concepts of the representational world. In addition, internal working models in attachment theory focus primarily on the content (i.e., positive versus negative) of representations of self and others and not on the structure of the cognitive schema. Although attachment theorists have forged links between a Piagetian stage of object permanence and the consolidation of internal working models of attachment (Bretherton, 1985; Main et al., 1985), they have not explored the implication of such a link for understanding aspects of the process of internalization in secure and insecure internal working models of attachment relationships. Different patterns of attachment not only involve differences in the content of internal working models but also differences in the structure of those models (e.g., degree of differentiation and integration), and it may be the structure of these models, more so than the content, that results in different capacities and potentials for adaptation. Thus, within specific attachment styles, internal working models may vary in the degree of differentiation, integration, and internalization (Diamond and Blatt, 1994; Levy et al., 1998). Even the concept of narrative "coherence" from the AAI scoring system (Main et al., 1985) is not linked to developmental processes and does not identify differences in the structure of representation. The concept of coherence of the narrative in the AAI is based on discourse usage as identified in linguistic analysis (e.g., Grice, 1975) such as adherence to or violation of four linguistic maxims (quality, quantity, relation, and manner).

Integrating Psychoanalytic and Attachment Theory
Perspectives on Representation

A recent formulation of personality development provides a potential basis for introducing a developmental perspective into attachment research and theory. Blatt and colleagues (Blatt, 1974; Blatt and Shichman, 1983; Blatt and Blass, 1990, 1995) propose a broad theoretical model of personality development involving a multidimensional dialectic interaction of two primary developmental lines of interpersonal relatedness and self-definition. They posit that psychological development involves two fundamental developmental tasks: (1) the establishment of the capacity to form stable, enduring, mutually satisfying, reciprocal interpersonal relationships and (2) the achievement of a differentiated, consolidated, stable, realistic, essentially positive identity. Normal development throughout the life cycle involves a complex, reciprocal transaction between these two developmental sequences. Meaningful and satisfying relationships contribute to the evolving concept of the self, and a new sense of self leads, in turn, to more mature levels of interpersonal relatedness (Blatt, 1974; Blatt and Shichman, 1983; Blatt and Blass, 1990, 1991, 1992; Blatt, 1990, 1995). The relatedness developmental line is characterized by concerns with trust, warmth, cooperation, and intimacy, while the self-definitional developmental line is characterized by concerns with autonomy, initiative, self-worth, and identity. Moreover, levels of personality and cognitive organization within each of these two developmental lines or sequences range from relatively undifferentiated and unintegrated to highly differentiated and integrated levels. These two developmental lines not only provide a basis for considering personality development, but they have particular relevance for the conceptualization of psychopathology. Distortions and exaggerated emphasis of either developmental line and the defensive avoidance of the other leads to particular configurations of psychopathology (Blatt and Shichman, 1983). Moreover, Blatt and Shichman (1983) contend that these two different configurations are related to several types of personality disorder behaviors. In their discussion, they posit that exaggerated and distorted emphasis on the interpersonal (or anaclitic development) is related to depression, hysteria, and dependent and borderline personalities. In contrast, the self-definitional (or introjective) developmental line is related to self-critical, guilty (introjective) depression, phallic narcissism, obsessive-compulsive, paranoid, schizoid, schizotypal, and overideational borderline personalities.

As indicated by attachment research, secure attachment involves both a capacity to establish affective bonds and to tolerate and benefit from separation. Secure attachment involves both increasingly mature levels of interpersonal relatedness and of autonomy and individuation as expressed in the capacity to both love and to work (Hazan and Shaver, 1990). Thus, secure attachment represents an integration of these two developmental lines and involves an integrated and coordinated development of the capacity for establishing mature levels of interpersonal relatedness and essentially positive and realistic senses of self. These capacities are hypothesized to derive from the degree of differentiation and integration of representations of self and others, which allows for a nuanced, contextual, and diverse understanding of one's experience, the complexity of others, and the social world.

The application of this cognitive developmental, object relations perspective to attachment theory could provide a broader elucidation of interpersonal functioning from relatively less to more adaptive manifestations within each of the insecure types, thus giving attachment theory broader application to both nonclinical and clinical populations. Recent theorizing has related the introjective and anaclitic developmental lines to avoidant and preoccupied attachment styles, respectively (Pilkonis, 1988; Blatt and Homann, 1992; Blatt and Maroudas, 1992; Levine and Tuber, 1993). For example, the interpersonal (or anaclitic) developmental line is characterized by exaggerated attempts to establish interpersonal relationships similar to anxious–ambivalent attachment with its fears of abandonment and compulsive careseeking. A number of studies have shown that anxious–ambivalent/preoccupied attachment is associated with the anaclitic/dependent type of depression, characterized by concerns with disruptions of interpersonal relations and fears of abandonment and loneliness. Avoidant attachment has been associated with an introjective/self-critical type of depression, characterized by concerns about loss of self-esteem and feelings of worthlessness, blame, and guilt (Kelly, Levy, and Blatt, 1994; Zuroff and Fitzpatrick, 1995).

Developmental Levels within Avoidant Attachment

Bartholomew's identification of two types of avoidant attachment (fearful and dismissive) may actually represent two developmental levels that can be differentiated within the avoidant insecure attachment style. Levy et al.'s (1998) study of the relationship between young adults' attachment styles and the content and structure of their mental representations of their parents found that the descriptions of parents by dismissively avoidant subjects, as compared to descriptions by fearfully avoidant subjects, were significantly less differentiated, less conceptually complex, and less elaborate (had fewer attributes). Though fearful avoidant subjects, in contrast, represented their parents as more malevolent and punitive, their descriptions were more differentiated and at a higher conceptual level than dismissive subjects; in fact, the descriptions given by fearful avoidant individuals were similar on these dimensions to those of secure subjects. Fearful avoidant individuals expressed significantly greater ambivalence when describing their parents than dismissively avoidant subjects, primarily because dismissive subjects described their parents in polarized terms as *either* highly idealized or as punitive, malevolent, and lacking warmth. The ambivalence displayed in the descriptions of parents by fearful avoidant individuals suggests that they have an increased acknowledgment or awareness of negative aspects of their feelings about their parents and an ability to tolerate contradiction in others. In contrast, the lack of ambivalence in the descriptions of parents of dismissing avoidant subjects suggests an avoidance of conflictual issues in their inability to acknowledge both positive and negative aspects of their parents—an essential step toward more differentiated and integrated representations. The descriptions of dismissing individuals have a one-sided polarized quality—either idealizing or denigrating, with relatively little complexity and expression of ambivalence. These findings are consistent with research on adult attachment that has found that avoidant subjects have more difficulty integrating both positive and negative qualities of romantic partners (Hazan and Shaver, 1987) and of early relationships with parents (Main et al., 1985). Additionally, Main et al., (1985), Kobak and Sceery (1988), Hazan and Shaver (1987), and others (Mikulincer et al., 1990; Simpson et al., 1992) all stress that dismissing avoidant subjects are unable to deal with emotions, particularly negative emotions. These findings are also congruent with previous research on mental representations that indicate that the complexity of representations of others allows for better tolerance and integration of negative feelings toward others (Diamond et al., 1990; Gruen and Blatt, 1990). The finding that secure and fearful individuals gave more articulated descriptions (i.e., had more attributes) indicates a greater capacity for emotional elaboration. Although fearfully avoidant subjects have more ambivalent and more negative representations of their parents, they appreciate the complexity of relationships and differentiate themselves and their parents more fully than do dismissively avoidant subjects. These findings suggest that dismissive avoidance is a less adaptive expression of avoidant attachment than fearful avoidance. Thus, these findings suggest a developmental differentiation within avoidant insecure attachment based on the degree of differentiation and integration of representations—fearful avoidant subjects appear to be developmentally more mature than dismissively avoidant subjects. Dismissive avoidance appears to represent a less integrated and adaptive expression of avoidant attachment style.

Developmental Levels Within Preoccupied Anxious–Ambivalent Attachment

Similar to the identification of two developmental levels of avoidant attachment, a differentiation appears possible within the preoccupied (anxious–ambivalent) style of attachment. Hazan and Shaver and Main and colleagues describe the anxious pattern of attachment as characterized by compulsive careseeking and a fear of abandonment. West and colleagues (West and Sheldon, 1988), primarily from a clinical perspective consistent with Bowlby's original formulations, discussed how a preoccupation with relatedness can be expressed as either compulsive careseeking or compulsive caregiving. They developed a self-report measure for these two insecure styles and for two other insecure patterns of insecure attachment (compulsive self-reliance and angry withdrawal). Compulsive careseeking, as described by Bowlby (1977), is characterized by urgent and frequent careseeking behaviors in order to maintain a sense of security. Bowlby (1977) hypothesized that this pattern develops from the infant's experience of an unreliable, unavailable, or unresponsive caregiver. Compulsive caregiving, in contrast, appears to reflect a more mature and integrated expression or higher developmental level of a preoccupied attachment style as compared to the less mature, unilateral, nonreciprocal, compulsive careseeking. Compulsive caregiving, on the other hand, is a pattern of attachment resulting from role-reversal, in which the child assumes the role of the caregiving parent. This pattern emerges out of an infant–caregiver relationship marked by the mother's need for symbiosis, in which the mother seeks to obtain need gratification by using her child as an attachment figure. The compulsive caregiver provides care in the way he or she wants to be cared for, and therefore, this style may have greater potential for establishing a sense of relatedness, eventually with reciprocity and mutuality. Compulsive careseekers, in contrast, seem less mature because they primarily seek unilateral relationships that provide contact, nurturance, gratification, support, approval, and acceptance from others. Schaffer (1993) found that compulsive careseekers reported significantly greater levels of dependency, self-criticism, and anxiety, as well as a lower level of self-efficacy than compulsive caregivers. Schaffer (1993) also found that compulsive caregivers, as compared to careseekers, have more adaptive forms of regulating affect. Specifically, compulsive careseeking attachment is associated with oral/somatic and sexual/ aggressive ways of affect regulation, while compulsive caregiving attachment is associated with cognitive and social/interpersonal efforts of affect regulation, suggesting that the latter group has access to more adaptive forms of affect regulation. Additionally, compulsive caregiving subjects, like secure subjects, were more successful at using interpersonal efforts to regulate affect and were generally more successful at modulating affect than compulsive careseekers. Schaffer also found that compulsive careseekers score higher than both compulsive caregivers and secure subjects on measures of alexithymia, indicating that compulsive careseekers may have diffi-culty differentiating and describing their feelings. Compulsive careseekers employ maladaptive action patterns and self-sacrificing defenses, while compulsive caregivers used more adaptive defenses. Thus, Schaffer's (1993) findings suggest a developmental continuum along the preoccupied/anxious–ambivalent spectrum, with compulsive caregiving attachment reflecting a higher developmental level of attachment as compared to compulsive careseeking attachment. Compulsive careseeking is characterized by the use of relationships primarily for the gratification of one's needs with little awareness of the other as a separate individual with needs of his or her own. Because of deficits in evocative constancy, compulsive careseekers are more reliant on the presence of attachment figures. In contrast, compulsive caregiving attachment reflects a relationship that is centered around the gratification of the needs of the other. In order to care for another, one must perceive and appreciate the needs of the other. In this respect, compulsive caregiving requires greater differentiation between self and other and thus represents a higher developmental level. Subsequent research should be directed toward comparing the mental representations of self and significant others of compulsive careseekers and compulsive caregivers.

Additional evidence for a developmental distinction within the anxious–ambivalent/preoccupied style comes from research by Blatt and colleagues on different types of depression. Blatt and colleagues (Blatt, D'Afflitti, and Quinlan, 1976) developed a questionnaire that measures anaclitic (dependent) and introjective (self-critical) tendencies (Depressive Experiences Questionnaire [DEQ], which assesses a broad range of feelings and beliefs regarding the self and interpersonal relationships. Specifically, three factors on the DEQ assess experiences of dependency, self-criticism, and efficacy. These factors have good levels of internal consistency and test–retest reliability and have been replicated in other samples (Zuroff, Quinlan, and Blatt, 1991). Numerous studies demonstrate the validity of the three factors (see Blatt and Zuroff, 1992, for a review).

Recently, Blatt and colleagues (Blatt et al., 1993) identified two subscales within the Dependency factor: (a) an anaclitic dependency or neediness subscale characterized by items that expressed concerns with feelings of helplessness, having fears and apprehensions about separateness and rejection and intense concerns about loss of gratification and experiences of frustration; and (b) a relatedness subscale characterized by feelings of sadness and loneliness in response to disruptions of a specific relationship. Anaclitic dependency or neediness had significantly greater correlations with independent measures of depression, while interpersonal concerns had significantly higher correlations with measures of self-esteem (Blatt et al., 1993). These

findings provide further evidence of a differentiation of several
levels of developmental maturity within the quality of interpersonal
relatedness.

Attachment Theory, Psychoanalysis, and Psychopathology

A major implication of these formulations is that an important differentiation can be made within attachment categories based on the level
or degree of differentiation and integration of the underlying mental
representations or internal working models. These representations
occur along a developmental continuum ranging from lower to higher
levels of organization. These formulations provide a useful framework
for understanding the quality of interpersonal relationships based on a
fuller integration of attachment processes and psychoanalytic developmental theories of personality development and psychopathology.

Variability in the degree of differentiation and integration of mental
representations within attachment categories suggests that each
category encompasses individuals with different levels of object
relations and adaptive potentials. A number of studies (Alexander,
1993; Alexander et al., 1993; Levy, 1993; Anderson and Alexander,
1994; Rosenstein and Horowitz, 1996) have found that borderline,
histrionic, and dependent personality disorders are related to a preoccupied attachment style. For example, Levy (1993) examined the
relationship between adult attachment styles, using Bartholomew's
self-report attachment measure, and personality disorders, using the
Millon Clinical Multiaxial Inventory, in seventy-five college students.
They found that preoccupied attachment was related to measures of
borderline, dependent, and passive-aggressive personality disorders.
Fearful avoidant attachment was related to avoidant and schizoid
personality disorder. Dismissing avoidant attachment was related to
narcissistic, antisocial and paranoid personality disorders. Securely
attached individual's reported less schizoid, borderline, antisocial,
avoidant, schizotypal and passive-aggressive traits. In a study of 60
hospitalized adolescents, Rosenstein and Horowitz (1996), using the
AAI, found that preoccupied attachment was associated with histrionic, borderline, schizotypal, and obsessive-compulsive disorder and
self-reported avoidant, anxious, and dysthymic personality traits on

the Millon Clinical Multiaxial Inventory-II. Dismissing attachment was associated with narcissistic and antisocial personality disorders, and self-reported narcissistic, antisocial, and paranoid personality traits. Alexander and colleagues (Alexander, 1993; Alexander et al., 1993; Anderson and Alexander, 1994) in a sample of 112 adult female incest survivors assessed the relationship between attachment and personality disorders using both the AAI and Bartholomew's structured interview and self-report as measures of attachment and the Millon Multiaxial Clinical Inventory-II (MCMI-II; Millon, 1987). Preoccupied attachment was associated with dependent, avoidant, self-defeating, and borderline personality disorder. Fearful avoidance was correlated with avoidant, self-defeating, and borderline personality disorder. Dismissing subjects reported the least distress, most likely due to their proclivity to suppress negative affect (Kobak and Sceery, 1988). In terms of the AAI, unresolved subjects were the most distressed and showed the greatest likelihood of avoidant, self-defeating, and borderline personality disorder.

Further research (Levy et al., in press; Ouimette and Klein, 1993; Ouimette et al., 1994) using the DEQ has also found that personality disorders are related to anaclitic (anxious attachment) and introjective (avoidant attachment) developmental lines. In an inpatient sample, they found that the anaclitic developmental line was significantly related to histrionic, dependent, and borderline features and significantly negatively correlated with schizoid features. The introjective developmental line was related to schizoid, schizotypal, narcissistic, and borderline features. In addition, the difference between the correlations of the anaclitic and introjective developmental lines were significant for schizoid, narcissistic, and dependent personality disorders. Ouimette and colleagues (Ouimette and Klein, 1993; Ouimette et al., 1994) reported similar results in both a college sample and outpatient sample.

The findings of these studies also suggest the value of conceptualizing degrees or developmental levels within attachment patterns. Within the anxious- ambivalent/preoccupied/emeshed pattern or anaclitic developmental line, borderline, histrionic, hysterical, dependent, and infantile individuals are all concerned with bonding and relatedness, however, these disorders represent a wide range of functioning. Likewise, within the introjective developmental line, fearful avoidant attachment is related to obsessive-compulsive, avoidant and schizoid personality disorders and dismissing avoidant attachment is related to narcissistic, antisocial and paranoid personality disorders. Again, as with disorders in the anaclitic developmental line, these disorders in the introjective developmental line represent a wide range of functioning. Thus, the degree of differentiation and integration or developmental level of representations may provide an important basis for making distinctions within attachment categories that helps explain the relationship of attachment classifications to various types and degrees of psychopathology (Blatt, 1995).

In contrast, investigations in the Ainsworth tradition have specifically rejected the concept of levels of attachment in favor of the view that everyone forms attachments and that individuals (and relationships) differ in terms of attachment quality. That is, some individuals are secure in their attachment while others are insecure avoidant or insecure preoccupied in their attachment. The findings cited above suggest that individuals differ, however, not only in terms of attachment quality or style, but also in the level or degree of differentiation of internal working models that underlie these attachment patterns. Differences in attachment styles should be based not only on the degree, quality, or strength of attachment, but also on the degree of differentiation and integration of mental representations or internal working models that underlie these attachment organizations.

In terms of representational systems, borderline pathology results from a lack of differentiation and integration of multiple and often disparate representations. Additionally, borderline patients have difficulties in evocative constancy, that is—the ability to evoke and sustain enduring representations of self and others, particularly during stressful moments. Evocative constancy is the capacity to sustain a coherent image of the object regardless of his or her perceptual or emotional availability (Adler and Buie, 1979; Blatt and Shichman, 1983; Blatt and Auerbach, 1988). Psychoanalytic theorists such as Mahler and Kernberg and others have linked borderline pathology to failures to resolve the rapprochement crisis, a developmental process that occurs with the consolidation of the capacity for evocative constancy. Thus, when a significant relationship is disrupted or threat ened, the borderline patient experiences the other not only as disinterested or unavailable, but often as completely lost. Disturbances in evocative constancy among borderline patients are also expressed in an inability to maintain a cohesive, effective sense of self in the face of criticism or rejection. Cognitive processes become fragmented, idiosyncratic, and illogical (Blatt and Auerbach, 1988). Many aspects of the symptomatic expression of borderline pathology center on the failure of evocative constancy, including the vacillation between clinging and repudiation of others; the polarized often horrific, images of self and other; a pervasive sense of emptiness. Borderline patients tend to feel irrevocably abandoned when others are unavailable or unresponsive, and these patients are unable to sustain a stable sense of self or a benign sense of other in the face of criticism or rejection. They have the propensity toward exaggerated emotional displays and incessant emotional demands in order to sustain contact with the object (Blatt and Auerbach, 1988). All the foregoing may function, as "an attempt to vivify experiences to compensate for deficits in evocative schema" (Blatt, 1995, p. 452).

In contrast people with hysterical, dependent, and infantile personality disorders are better able than borderline individuals to evoke and maintain representations of self and others, however, these representations are not easily maintained and often feel tenuous. The infantile and dependent individuals are concerned about being cared for, often in terms of concrete aspects of the relationship. At a higher developmental level, hysterical individuals are concerned about establishing mutual relationships—wanting to love as well as be loved—and therefore are often concerned with the experiences and feelings of others.

The integration of psychoanalytic concepts with attachment theory enables us to view attachment styles not just as static, separate, and discrete types or categories, but also as based on the level of differentiation and integration of the underlying representational system that occurs along a developmental continuum ranging from lower to higher levels of organization. These formulations derive from an integration of attachment processes and psychoanalytic developmental theories of psychopathology.

Conclusions

Attachment theory and psychoanalysis (particularly object relations theory) can reciprocally inform and facilitate each other's development. Attachment theory and research provides a powerful and valuable heuristic framework for conducting psychoanalytic research, testing psychoanalytic hypotheses, and enriching the perspective of psychoanalytic clinicians and investigators. And conversely, psychoanalysis can contribute to attachment theory with concepts such as developmental levels of representation, thereby placing attachment theory in a broader theoretical context. This integration of attachment and psychoanalytic developmental theory provides a broad-ranging theoretical model of personality development and psychopathology across a wide developmental spectrum. Thus, psychoanalytic theory and research can enrich, and be enriched in turn, by attachment theory and research in understanding normal and disrupted developmental processes. Attachment theory provides a useful framework for the testing of psychoanalytic ideas, while psychoanalytic theory provides a broader elucidation of internal working models. The integration of these two bodies of knowledge can enrich our understanding of personality development (Blatt, Auerbach, and Levy, 1997) and psychopathology (Levy, 1993; Diamond et al., 1998) as well as the therapeutic process (Blatt et al., 1996; Fonagy et al., 1996; Blatt, Auerbach, and Levy, 1997; Slade, in press).

REFERENCES

Adler, G. & Buie, D. H. (1979), Aloneness and borderline psychopathology: The possible relevance of developmental issues. *Internat. J. Psychoanal.* 60:83–96.

Ainsworth, M. S. (1969), Object relations, dependency, and attachment: Theoretical review of infant–mother relationship. *Devel. Psychol.*, 40:969–1025.

———— Bell, S. M. & Stayton, D. J. (1971), Individual differences in strange situation behavior of one-year-olds. In: *The Origins of Human Social Relations,* ed., H. R. Schaffer. New York: Academic Press, pp. 17–57.

———— ———— ———— (1974), Infant-mother attachment and social behavior: Socialization as a product of reciprocal response to signals. In: *The Integration of a Child into a Social World,* ed. M. P. M. Richards. London: Cambridge University Press, pp. 99–135.

———— Blehar, M. C., Waters, E. and Wall, S. (1978), *Patterns of Attachment.* Hillsdale, NJ: Lawrence Erlbaum Associates.

Alexander, P. C. (1993), The differential effects of abuse characteristics and attachment in the prediction of long-term effects of sexual abuse. *J. Interpers. Violence,* 8:346–362.

———— & Anderson, C. L. (1994), An attachment approach. *Psychotherapy,* 31:665–675.

Bartholomew, K. (1989), *Attachment styles in young adults: Implications of self-concept and interpersonal functioning.* Unpublished Doctoral Dissertation. Stanford University, Palo Alto, CA.
————— (1990), Avoidance of intimacy: An attachment perspective. *J. Soc. & Personal Relationships,* 7:147–178.
————— & Horowitz, L. (1991), Attachment styles among young adults: A four category model of attachment. *J. Personal. & Soc. Psychol.,* 61:226–241.
————— & Shaver, P. R. (1998), Measures of attachment: Do they all converge? In: *Attachment Theory and Close Relationships,* ed. J. A. Simpson and W. S. Rholes. New York: Guilford, pp. 25–45.
Beres, D. & Joseph, E. (1970), The concept of mental representation in psychoanalysis. *Internat. J. Psycho-Anal.,* 51:1–9.
Blatt, S. J. (1974), Levels of object representation in anaclitic and introjective depression. *The Psychoanalytic Study of the Child,* 29:107–157. New Haven, CT: Yale University Press.
————— (1990), Interpersonal relatedness and self-definition: Two personality configurations and their implications for psychopathology and psychotherapy. In: *Repression and Dissociation: Implications for Personality Theory, Psychopathology and Health,* ed. J. L. Singer. Chicago, IL: University of Chicago Press, pp. 299–335.
————— (1991), Cognitive morphology of psychopathology. *J. Nervous & Mental Dis.,* 179:449–458.
————— (1995), Representational structures in psychopathology. In: *Representation, Emotion, and Cognition in Developmental Psychopathology,* ed. D. Cicchetti and S. Toth. Rochester, NY: University of Rochester Press, pp. 1–33.
————— & Auerbach, J. S. (1988), Differential cignitive disturbances in three types of "borderline" patients. *J. Personality Disorders,* 2:198–211.
————— and Blass, R. B. (1990), Attachment and separateness: A dialectic model of the products and processes of development throughout the life cycle. *The Psychoanalytic Study of the Child,* 45:107–127. New Haven, CT: Yale University Press.
————— and ————— (1995), Relatedness and self-definition: A dialectic model of personality development. In: *Development and Vulnerabilities in Close Relationships,* G. G. Noam and K. W. Fischer. Hillsdale, NJ: Lawrence Erlbaum Associates, pp. 309–338.
————— & Homann, E. (1992), Parent–child interaction in the etiology of dependent and self-critical depression. *Clin. Psychol. Rev.,* 12:47–92.
————— & Lerner, H. D. (1983), The psychological assessment of object representation. *J. Personal. Assess.,* 47:7–28.
————— & Maroundas, C. (1992), Convergence among psychoanalytic and cognitive-behavioral theories of depression. Psychoanal. Psychol. 9:157–190.
————— & Shichman, S. (1983), Two primary configurations of psychopathology. *Psychoanal. & Contemp. Thought,* 6:187–254.
————— & Zuroff, D. (1992), Interpersonal relatedness and self-definition: Two prototypes for depression. Clinical Psychol. Rev., 12:527–562.
————— D'Afflitti, J. P., Quinlan, D. M. (1976), Experiences of depression in normal young adults. *J. Abnormal Psychol.,* 85:383–389.
————— ————— & Levy, K. N. (1997), Mental representations in personality development, psychopathology, and the therapeutic process. *General Psychology Review,* 1:351–374.

────── Stayner, D. A. Auerbach, J. S. & Behrends, R. (1996), Change in object and self representations in long-term intensive inpatient treatment of seriously disturbed adolescents and young adults. *Psychiatry,* 59:82–107.

────── Zohar, A. H., Quinlan, D. M., Zuroff, D. C. & Mongrain, M. (1995), Subscales within the dependency factor of the depressive experiences question-naire. *J. Personal. Assess.,* 64:319–339.

Borman, E. & Cole, H. (1993), A comparison of three measures of adult attachment. Poster presented at the biennial meeting of the Society for Research in Child Development, New Orleans, LA.

Bornstein, R. F., Galley, D. J. & Leone, D. R. (1986), Parental representations and orality. *J. Personal. Assess.,* 50:80–89.

────── Leone, D. R., & Galley, D. J. (1988), Rorschach measures of oral dependence and the internalized self-representation in normal college students. *J. Personal. Assess.,* 52:648–657.

────── ────── & ────── (1990), Construct validity of Blatt's measure of qualitative and structural dimensions of object representations: Test–retest stability of parental contact. *J. Soc. Behav. & Personal.,* 6:641–649.

Bowlby, J. (1944), Forty-four juvenile thieves: Their characters and home-life (I). *Internat. J. Psychoanal.* 25:19–53.

────── (1969), *Attachment and Loss: Vol 1. Attachment.* New York: Basic Books.

────── (1973), *Attachment and Loss: Vol. 2. Separation,* New York: Basic Books.

────── (1977), The making and breaking of affectional bonds: 1. Etiology and psychopathology in light of attachment theory. *Brit. J. Psychiat.* 130:201–210.

────── (1979), *The Making and Breaking of Affectional Bonds.* New York: Tavistock Publications.

────── (1980), *Attachment and Loss: Vol. 3. Loss: Sadness and Depression.* New York: Basic Books.

────── (1988), *A Secure Base.* New York: Basic Books.

Brennan, K. A., Shaver, P. R., and Tobey, A. E. (1991), Attachment styles, gender, and parental problem drinking. *J. Soc. & Personal Relation.,* 8:451–466.

────── & Shaver, P. R. (1994), Dimensions of adult attachment, affect regulation, and romantic relationship functioning. *Personal. & Soc. Psychol. Bull., 21,* 267–283.

Bretherton, I. (1985), Attachment theory: Retrospect and prospect. *Monographs of the Soc. Res. Child Dev.,* 50, (1 & 2), Serial No. 209, 3–35.

────── (1987), New perspectives on attachment relations: Security, communication, and internal working models. In: *Handbook of Infant Development,* ed. J. Osofoky. New York: Wiley, pp. 1061–1100.

Collins, N. L. & REad, S. J. (1990), Adult attachment, working models, and relation-ship quality in dating couples. *J. Personal. & Social Psychol.,* 58:644–663.

Crowell, J. A. & Feldman, S. S. (1988), Mothers' internal models of relationships and children's behavioral and developmental status: A study of mother–child interac-tion. *Child Develop.,* 59:1273–1285.

────── Treboux, D. & Waters, E. (1993), *Alternatives to the AAI? Self-reports of attachment style and relationship with mothers and partners.* Poster presented at the biennial meeting of the Society for Research in Child Development, New Orleans, LA.

────── Fraley, R. C. & Shaver, P. R. (1999), Measurement of adult attachment. In: Handbook of Attachment, ed. J. Cassidy & P. R. Shaver. New York: Guilford Press.

Diamond, D. & Blatt, S. J. (1994), Internal working models of attachment and psychoanalytic theories of the representational world: A comparison and critique. In: *Attachment in Adults: Clinical and Developmental Perspectives*, ed. M. B. Sperling and W. H. Berman. New York: Guilford Press, pp. 72–97.

—— Kaslow, N., Coonerty, S. & Blatt, S. J. (1990), Changes in separation–individuation and intersubjectivity in long-term treatment. *Psychoanal. Psychol.*, 7:363–397.

—— Blatt, S. J., Stayner, D. & Kaslow, N. (1992), Differentiation, cohesion, and relatedness of self and other representations: A developmental scale. Unpublished manuscript.

Egeland, B. & Farber, E. A. (1984), Infant–mother attachment: Factors related to its development and changes over time. *Child Develop.*, 88:753–771.

Elicker, J., Englund, M. & Sroufe, L. A. (1993), Predicting peer competence and peer relationships in childhood from early parent–child relationships. In: *Family–Peer Relationships: Modes of Linkage*, ed. R. D. Parke & G. W. Ladd. Hillsdale, NJ: Lawrence Erlbaum Associates, pp. 77–106.

Emde, R. N. (1983), The prerepresentational self and its affective core. *The Psychoanalytic Study of the Child*. New Haven, CT: Yale University Press.

Erikson, M. F., Sroufe, L. A. and Egeland, B. (1985), The relationship between quality of attachment and behavior problems in pre-school in a high risk sample. In: *Growing Points in Attachment*, ed. I. Bretherton & E. Waters. *Monographs of the Society for Research in Child Development*, 50:147–166.

Fairbairn, W. R. D. (1952), *Psychoanalytic Studies of the Personality*. London: Routledge & Kegan Paul.

Feeney, B. C. & Kirkpatrick, L. A. (1996), Effects of adult attachment and presence of romantic partners on physiological responses to stress. *J. Personal. & Social Psychol.*, 70:255–270.

Feeney, J. A. & Noller, P. (1990), Attachment style as a predictor of adult romantic relationships. *J. Personal. & Social Psychol.*, 58:281–291.

—— Noller, P. & Hanrahan, M. (1994), Assessing adult attachment: Developments in the conceptualization of security and insecurity. In: *Attachment in Adults*, ed. M. B. Sperling and W. H. Berman. New York: Guilford, pp. 128–154.

Fonagy, P., Leigh, T., Steele, M., Steele, H., Kennedy, R., Mattoon, G., Target, M. & Gerber, A. (1996), The relation of attachment status, psychiatric classification and response to psychotherapy. *J. Consult. & Clinical Psychol.*, 64:22–31.

Fraley, R. C. & Shaver, P. R. (1998), Airport separations: A naturalistic study of adult attachment dynamics in separating couples. J. Personal. & Social Psychol., 75:1198–1212.

Freud, S. (1914), On narcissism: An introduction. *Standard Edition*, 14:73–102. London: Hogarth Press, 1957.

George, C. Kaplan, N. & Main, M. (1985), The Berkeley Adult Attachment Interview. Unpublished manuscript, Department of Psychology, University of California, Berkeley.

Goldberg, S., Perrutton, M. & Minde, K. (1986), Maternal behavior and attachment in low birth-weight twins and singletons. *Child Develop.*, 57:34–46.

Grice, H. P. (1975), Logic and conversation. In: *Syntax and Semantics, Vol. 3*, ed. P. Cole & J. L. Moran., New York: Academic Press, pp. 41-58.

Griffin, D. W. & Bartholomew, K. (1994a), The metaphysics of measurement: The case of adult attachment. In: *Advances in Personal Relationships*, K. Bartholomew & D. Perlman. London: Jessica Kingsley, pp. 17–52.

———— Bartholomew, K. (1994b), Models of the self and other: Fundamental dimensions underlying measures of adult attachment. *J. Personal. & Soc. Psychol.* 67:430–445.

Grossmann, K. E. & Grossmann, K. (1991), Attachment quality as an organizer of emotional behavioral responses in a longitudinal perspective. In: *Attachment Across the Life Cycle*, ed. C. M. Parkes, J. Stevenson-Hinde, & P. Marris. London: Tavistock/Routledge, pp. 93–114.

Grossman, K., Grossman, K. E., Spangler, G., Suss, G. & Unznor, L. (1985), Maternal sensitivity and newborns' orientation responses as related to quality of attachment in Northern Germany. In: *Growing Points of Attachment Theory and Research*, ed. I. Bretherton & J. E. Waters. *Monogr. Soc. Research in Child Development*, 50 (1–2, serial #209), pp. 233–256.

Gruen, R. & Blatt, S. J. (1990), Changes in self- and object representation during long-term dynamically oriented treatment. *Psychoanal. Psychol.*, 7:399–422.

Guntrip, H. (1971), *Psychoanalytic Theory, Therapy, and the Self*. New York: Basic Books.

Hazan, C. & Hutt, M. (1991), The process of relinquishing parents as attachment figures. Paper presented at the biennial meetings of the Society for Research in Child Development, Seattle, WA, April.

———— & Shaver, P. R. (1987), Romantic love conceptualized as an attachment process. *J. Personal. & Soc. Psychol.*, 52:511–524.

———— & ———— (1990), Love and work: An attachment–theoretical perspective. *J. Personal. & Soc. Psychol.*, 59:270–280.

———— & Shaver, P. R. (1994), Attachment as an organizational framework for research on close relationships. *Psycholog. Inq.*, 5:1–22.

Horowitz, L. M., Rosenberg, S. E. & Bartholemew, K. (1993), Interpersonal problems, attachment styles, and outcome in brief dynamic psychotherapy. *J. Consulting & Clin. Psychol.*, 61:549–560.

Horowitz, M. J. (1977), Structure and processes of change. In: *Hysterical Personality*, ed. M. J. Horowitz. New York: Aronson.

Isabella, R. A. & Belsky, J. (1991), Interactional synchrony and origins of infant–mother attachment: A replication study. *Child Devel.*, 62:373–384.

Jacobson, E. (1964), *The Self and the Object World*. New York: International Universities Press.

Karen, R. (1994), *Becoming Attached*. New York: Warner Books.

Kelly, K. M., Levy, K. N. & Blatt, S. J. (1996), *Attachment Styles and Depression*. New research presented at the 1996 American Psychiatric Association Annual Meeting, New York, NY, May.

———— (1976), *Object Relations Theory and Clinical Psychoanalysis*. New York: Aronson.

———— & Hazan, C. (1994), Attachment styles and close relationships: A four-year prospective study. *Personal Relations,*, 1:123–142.

Kirkpatrick, L. A. & Davis, K. E. (1994), Attachment style, gender, and relationship stability: A longitudinal analysis. *J. Personal. & Social Psychol.*, 66:502–512.

Kobak, R. R. & Sceery, A. (1988), Attachment in late adolescence: Working models, affect regulation, and representation of self and others. *Child Devel.*, 59:135–146.

Levine, L. V. & Tuber, S. B. (1993), Measures of mental representation: Clinical and theoretical considerations. *Bull. Menn. Clinic*, 57:69–87.

Levy, K. N. (1993), *Adult Attachment Styles and Personality Pathology*. New research presented at the 1993 American Psychiatric Association Annual Meeting, San Francisco, CA, May.

——— Edell, W. S., Blatt, S. J., Becker, D. F., Quinlan, D. M., Kolligian, J. & McGlashan, T. H. (in press), Two configurations of psychopathology: The relationship of dependency, anaclitic neediness, and self-criticism to personality pathology. *J. Personality*.

——— Blatt, S. J. & Shaver, P. R. (1998), Attachment styles and parental representations. *J. Personal. & Social Psychol.*, 74:407–419.

Litchenberg, J. (1985), Response: In search of the elusive baby. *Psychoanal. Inq.*, 5:621–648.

Main, M. & Hesse, E. (1990), Parents' unresolved traumatic experiences are related to infant disorganized status: Is frightened and/or frightening parental behavior the linking mechanism? In: *Attachment in the Preschool Years: Theory, Research and Intervention*, ed. M. T. Greenberg, D. Cicchetti, & E. M. Cummings. Chicago: University of Chicago Press, pp. 161–184.

——— & Solomon, J. (1990), Procedures for identifying infants as disorganized/disoriented during the Ainsworth Strange Situation. In: *Attachment in the Preschool Years: Theory, Research and Intervention*, ed. M. T. Greenberg, D. Cicchetti & E. M. Cummings. Chicago: University of Chicago Press, pp. 95–124.

——— Kaplan, N. & Cassidy, J. (1985), Security in infancy, childhood, and adulthood: A move to the level of representation. *Monogr. Soc. for Res. Child Devel.* 50, (1 and 2), Serial No. 209, 66–104.

Mahler, M., Pine, F. & Bergman, A. (1975), *The Psychological Birth of the Human Infant*. New York: Basic Books.

Main, M. & Cassidy, J. (1988), Categories of response with the parent at age six: Predicted from infant attachment classifications and stable over a one month period. *Devel. Psychol.*, 24:415–426.

——— & Goldwyn, R. (1985), Adult attachment scoring and classification system. Unpublished scoring manual. Department of Psychology, University of California, Berkeley.

Matas, L., Arend, R. & Sroufe, L. A. (1978), Continuity of adaptation in the second year: The relationship between quality of attachment and later competence. *Child Devel.*, 49:547–556.

Mikulincer, M. & Nachshon, O. (1991), Attachment styles and patterns of self-disclosure. *J. Personal. & Soc. Psychol.*, 61:321–331.

——— Florian, V. & Tolmacz, R. (1990), Attachment style and fear of personal death: A case study of affect regulation. *J. Personality & Social Psychol.*, 58:273–280.

Millon, T. (1981), *Disorders of Personality: DSM-III, Axis II*. New York: Wiley.

——— (1987), *Millon Clinical Multiaxial Inventory-II Manual*. Minneapolis, MN: National Computer Systems.

Ouimette, P. C., & Klein, D. N. (1993), The convergence of psychoanalytic and cognitive-behavioral theories of depression: A review of the empirical literature and new data on Blatt's and Beck's models. In: *Empirical Studies of Psychoanalytic Theories, Vol. 4*, ed. R. Bornstein & J. Masling, ??.

———— Klein, D. N., Anderson, R., Riso, L. P. & Lizardi, H. (1994), Relationship of sociotropy/autonomy and dependency/self-criticism to DSM-III-R personality disorders. *J. Abnormal Psychol.,* 103:743–749.

Patterson, A. & Moran, G. (1988), Attachment theory, personality development, and psychotherapy. *Clinical Psychol. Rev.,* 8:611–636.

Pederson, D. R., Moran, G., Sitko, C., Campbell, K., Ghesquire, K. & Acton, H. (1990), Maternal sensitivity and the security of infant–mother attachment: A Q-Sort Study. *Child Devel.,* 61:1974–1983.

Piaget, J. (1952), *The Origins of Intelligence in Children.* New York: International Universities Press.

Pilkonis, P. A. (1988), Personality prototypes among depressives: Themes of dependency and autonomy. *J. Personality Disorders,* 2:144–152.

Quinlan, D. M., Blatt, S. J., Chevron, E. S. & Wein, S. J. (1992), Parental descriptions: Benevolence, punitiveness, and ambition. *J. Personal. Assess.,* 59:340–351.

Rholes, W. S., Simpson, J. A. & Blakely, B. S. (1995), Adult attachment styles and mothers' relationships with their young children. *Personal Relationships,* 2:35–54.

Rosenstein, D. S. & Horowitz, H. A. (19??), Adolescent attachment and psychopathology. *J. Consulting & Clinical Psychol.,* 64:244–253.

Rothbard, J. C. & Shaver, P. R. (1994), Continuity of attachment across the life span. In: *Attachment in Adults: Clinical and Developmental Perspectives,* ed. M. B. Sperling & W. H. Berman. New York: Guilford Press, pp. 31–71.

Sandler, J. & Rosenblatt, B. (1972), The concept of the representational world. *The Psychoanalytic Study of the Child,* 17:128–145. New York: International Universities Press.

Schaffer, C. E. (1993), The role of adult attachment in the experience and regulation of affect. Unpublished doctoral dissertation, Yale University.

Scharfe, E. & Bartholomew, K. (1994), Reliability and stability of adult attachment patterns. *Personal Relationships,* 1:23–43.

———— & Clark, C. L. (1994), The psychodynamics of adult romantic attachment. In: *Empirical perspectives on object relations theories,* ed. R. F. Bornstein & J. M. Masling. Washington, D.C.: American Psychological Association, pp. 105–156.

———— & Hazan, C. (1987), Being lonely, falling in love: Perspectives from attachment theory. *J. Soc. Behav. & Personal.,* 2:105–124.

———— & ———— (1993), Adult romantic attachment: Theory and evidence. In: *Advances in Personal Relationships, Vol. 4,* ed. D. Perlman & W. Jones. London: Jessica Kingsley, pp. 29–70.

———— ———— & Bradshaw, D. (1988), Love as attachment: The integration of three behavioral systems. In: *The Psychology of Love,* ed. R. J. Sternberg & M. Barnes. New Haven, CT: Yale University Press, pp. 68–99.

Shaver, P. R., Belsky, J. & Brennan, K. A. (under review), Comparing measures of adult attachment: An examination of interview and self-report methods. *Personal Relationships.*

Simpson, J. A. (1990), Influence of attachment styles on romantic relationships. *J. Personality & Social Psychol.,* 59:971–980.

———— Rholes, W. S. & Nelligan, J. S. (1992), Support seeking and support giving within couples in an anxiety-provoking situation: The role of attachment styles. *J. Personal. & Soc. Psychol.,* 60:434–446.

Slade, A. (in press), Attachment theory and research: Implications for theory and practice of individual psychotherapy. In: *Handbook of Attachment Theory and Research*, ed. J. Cassidy & P. Shaver. New York: Guilford Press.

———— & Aber, J. L. (1992), Attachments, drives, and development: Conflicts and convergences in theory. In: *The Interface of Psychoanalysis and Psychology*, ed. J. Barron, M. Eagle, & D. Wolitsky. Washington, D.C.: American Psychological Association, pp. 154–185.

Smith, P. B., & Pederson, D. R. (1988), Maternal sensitivity and patterns of infant–mother attachment. *Child Devel.*, 59:1097–1101.

Sperling, M. B. & Berman, W. H. (1991), An attachment classification of desperate love. J. Personal. Assess., 56:45–55.

Sroufe, L. A. (1983), Infant-caregiver attachment and patterns of adaptation in the preschool: The roots of competence and maladaption. *Minnesota Symposium in Child Psychology*, ed. M. Perlmutter. 16:41–83.

———— & Fleeson, J. (1986), Attachment and the construction of relationships. In: *Relationships and Development*, ed. W. W. Harup & Z. Rubin. Hillsdale, NJ: Lawrence Erlbaum Associates, pp. 51–71.

Stern, D. (1985), *The Interpersonal World of the Infant*. New York: Basic Books.

van IJzendoorn, M. H. (1995), Adult attachment representations, parental responsiveness, and infant attachment: A meta-analysis on the predictive validity of the AAI. *Psycholog. Bull.*, 117:387–403.

Waters, E., Wippman, & Sroufe, L. A. (1979), Attachment, positive affect, and competence in the peer group: Two studies in construct validation. *Child Devel.*, 50:821–829.

———— Merrick, S. K., Albersheim, W. & Treboux, D. (1995), *Attachment security from infancy to early adulthood: A 20-year longitudinal study*. Poster presented at the biennial meeting of the society for Research in Child Development, Indianapolis, IN.

Werner, H. (1948), *Comparative Psychology of Mental Development*. New York: International Universities Press.

West, M. & Sheldon, A. E. R. (1988), Classification of pathological attachment patterns in adults. *J. Personality Disorders*, 2:153–159.

Winnicott, D. W. (1960), The theory of the parent–infant relationship. In: *The Maturational Processes and the Facilitating Environment*, ed. ?? New York: International Universities Press, pp. 37–55.

———— (1965), *The Maturational Processes and the Facilitating Environment*. New York: International Universities Press.

Zuroff, D. C. & Fitzpatrick, D. K. (1995), Depressive personality styles: Implications for adult attachment. *Personality and Individual Differences*, 18:253–365.

———— Quinlan, D. M. & Blatt, S. J. (1990), Psychometric properties of the DEQ. *J. Personality Assessment*, 55:65–72.

Department of Psychiatry
The New York Hospital-Cornell Medical Center
21 Bloomingdale Road
White Plains, NY 10605

The Two-Person Unconscious: Intersubjective Dialogue, Enactive Relational Representation, and the Emergence of New Forms of Relational Organization

KARLEN LYONS-RUTH, Ph.D.

R ECENT PSYCHOANALYTIC THEORY HAS MOVED INCREASINGLY toward a relational, intersubjective, and social–constructivist stance. In this view the psychoanalytic encounter is seen as mutually coconstructed between two active participants, with the subjectivities of both patient and analyst contributing to the form and content of the dialogue that emerges between them (McLaughlin, 1991; Hoffman, 1992; Ogden, 1994). The current emphasis in analytic writing on the importance of enactments in the treatment situation attempts to keep the lens focused squarely on the point of contact between the two analytic participants and on the form of the implicit transactions that emerge between them (e.g., Ogden, 1994). Clinical descriptions acknowledge the active contributions of both partners to the coconstruction of the enactment, even though the primary clinical interest may be in those features of the enactment that echo problematic aspects of the patient's interactions with other important people (Jacobs, 1991; Hoffman, 1992). Enactments have been viewed as

Dr. Lyons-Ruth is an Associate Professor at Harvard Medical School and Co-Director of Academic Training in Child Psychology at the Cambridge Hospital.

This paper is an elaboration of Working Paper 3 (K. Lyons-Ruth) of the Change Process Study Group of Boston (Jeremy Nahum, Chair).

important opportunities to gain a window on unconscious motivations and meanings held by the patient that have not been previously recognized or articulated (McLaughlin, 1991).

In this shift to a more fluid and mutual view of therapeutic process, the need for a psychoanalytic model of development has increasingly been questioned (e.g., Mitchell, 1988). Converging pressures on psychoanalytic theories of mind and of development have come from the increasing sophistication of both behavioral and neuroscientific research. New findings regarding the development and organization of mind, brain, and behavior have outstripped the pace of change in psychoanalytic theory, further undermining the credibility of older developmental models. In contrast to these changes that have fostered scepticism about the role of developmental theory, longitudinal attachment research has provided recent consistent support for the view that important dimensions of relational behavior are grounded in relational history. This emerging developmental research base supports the continued relevance of developmental history to psychoanalytic process and the concomitant need to refashion a psychoanalytic metatheory that is consistent both with the new research base and with a more fluid, mutual, and constructivist view of relational change in adulthood.

The initial questions that led to the concerns in this paper were questions taken as a focus by the Process of Change Study Group of Boston, namely: what are the noninterpretive mechanisms of change that operate in the psychoanalytic situation, and how might the study of development illuminate these mechanisms of change? These questions are more directly addressed in related papers (Boston Process of Change Study Group, 1998; Stern et al., 1998). In struggling with these questions, however, it became apparent that to consider how noninterpretive mechanisms lead to change, one also has to grapple with the issue of what changes.

Psychoanalysis has always been concerned with understanding the organization of meaning, with affects viewed as the central guides and directors of meaning. New research is now pressing psychoanalytically oriented scholars to expand accounts of how meaning systems are organized to include implicit or procedural forms of knowing. Procedural knowing refers to knowing how to do something and how to behave adaptively, rather than knowing information or images that can be consciously recalled and recounted (Cohen and Squire, 1980). The organization of memory and meaning in the implicit or enactive domain only becomes manifest in the doing. In accord with the current psychoanalytic interest in enactments in psychoanalytic treatment, I will refer to "knowing how to do" as enactive representation (see also Bruner, Olver, and Greenfield, 1966).

The central postulates of this paper will be (1) that much of our relational experience is represented in an implicit procedural or enactive form that is unconscious, though not necessarily dynamically unconscious; (2) that in both development and psychoanalysis, the increasing integration and articulation of new enactive "procedures for being with" destabilize existing enactive organization and serve as a primary engine of change; and (3) that enactive procedures become more articulated and integrated through participation in more coherent and collaborative forms of intersubjective interaction. Put another way, at the level of unconscious enactive procedures, the medium *is* the message; that is, the organization of meaning is implicit in the organization of the enacted relational dialogue and does not require reflective thought or verbalization to be, in some sense, known. In accord with infant observers such as Beebe and Lachmann (1994), enactive representation is viewed here as the earliest medium through which the "shadow of the object" becomes part of the "unthought known" of the infant's early experience (Bollas, 1987).

This paper will attempt to make more explicit a model of the development and change of enactive relational procedures that is consistent both with recent psychoanalytic literature and with recent findings in attachment research, early parent–infant interaction, cognitive neuroscience, and nonlinear dynamic systems theory. Attachment research has concentrated on describing and validating a range of organized strategies of caregiver–infant interaction around attachment needs that are represented by the infant by the end of the first year. More recent work has extended these descriptions of the infant's enactive representations around attachment needs to include the parent's corresponding enactive strategies for ways of responding to an interview about his or her own early attachment-related experiences. Although the details of these patterns of enactive relational representation in the realm of attachment experiences are important in themselves, they have been well described in the literature and will not be reviewed here (see Bretherton, 1988; Main, 1993; Lyons-Ruth and Jacobvitz, 1999). Instead, the focus of this paper will be on the implications of such enduring attachment-oriented enactive relational procedures for a general developmental–psychoanalytic theory of relational process and enactive representation. Attachment research has provided the most extensive empirical basis for this synthesis, but work on early face-to-face interaction and work on context-sensitive models of brain development and cognitive development, as well as research on adult cognition, also contribute to the emergence of the model.

Because it seems premature to rigidify a set of terms for describing this new conceptual territory, I will refer interchangeably to enactive representations, relational procedures, or implicit relational control systems. I use the term *representation* in relation to enactive knowing because, in keeping with prior psychoanalytic insights, this form of representation preserves knowledge of the affective-perceptual and spatio-temporal contingencies in the environment. I will also use *implicit* and *unconscious* interchangeably here to refer to the nondynamic procedural unconscious.

A central contention of this paper is that enactive knowing develops and changes by processes that are intrinsic to this system of representation and that do not rely on translation of procedures into reflective (symbolized) knowledge. This is not to contend that translating enactive knowledge into words may not be an important therapeutic tool or developmental step; it *is* to contend that development does not proceed only or primarily by moving from procedural coding to symbolic coding (*or* from primary to secondary process *or* from *pre*verbal to verbal forms of thought). Procedural forms of representation are not infantile but are intrinsic to human cognition at all ages and underlie many forms of skilled action, including intimate social interaction.

The elaboration of symbolic forms of thought, including both images and words, contains the potential to contribute to the reorganization of enactive knowing. However, I would contend that retranscription of implicit relational knowing into symbolic knowing is laborious, is not intrinsic to the affect-based relational system, is never completely accomplished, and is not how developmental change in implicit relational knowing is generally accomplished. Rather, I would argue that procedural systems of relational knowing develop in parallel with symbolic systems, as separate systems with separate governing principles. Procedural systems influence and are influenced by symbolic systems through multiple cross-system connections, but these influences are necessarily incomplete. Furthermore, enactive relational knowing is grounded in goal-directed action, along with the affective evaluations guiding that action, and so is likely to exert as much or more influence on how symbolic systems are elaborated as symbolic systems exert on how relational systems are elaborated (see Anderson, 1982; Schachter and Moscovitch, 1984; Damascio, 1994).

I sketch the outlines of a theory of psychoanalytic and developmental change based on unconscious or implicit enactive representation and patient–therapist transactions rather than on symbolized meaning and interpretation. This focus on the two- person process is intended to establish a theoretical framework through which long-standing clinical insights on the interplay of affect, conflict, defense, and resistance can be further extended into a two-person realm and given a scientifically credible developmental base. Although constructs of motivation and, to some extent, affect are not dealt with extensively here, they are intrinsic to any theory of enactive representation, and the current framework is intended to augment, not replace, the extensive literature on affect and motivation in analytic treatment. Similarly, many points of interface where the model described in this paper might converge with or complement self psychological or conflict models of intrapsychic organization are not made explicit here. Instead, the paper focuses on extending our conceptualization of the transactional space and its representational forms in development and in psychoanalytically oriented treatment.

The paper is divided into two parts. The first section focuses on the two-person dialogue in early development. Three central implications of current attachment research are highlighted. First, more flexible and inclusive enactive representations emerge from more collaborative forms of parent–child dialogue. Second, adult neuroscience converges with infant research to confirm the separate and dissociable status of conscious symbolized knowledge and nonsymbolized implicit or procedural knowing throughout the lifespan. Third, prior to the outset of symbol use, the infant's implicit relational procedures include indicators of conflict and defense that are tied to particular restrictions or distortions in the parent–infant affective dialogue.

The second section of the paper explores noninterpretive mechanisms of change in implicit relational control systems. The developmental models of Fischer (1980) and Case (1991) are reviewed which emphasize the context-dependent and fractionated nature of the development of skilled behavior, in both relational and nonrelational domains. Most importantly, Fischer and Case elaborate developmental models of how more complex control systems are elaborated from infancy to adulthood by coordinating enactive procedures with one another to form progressively more flexible and inclusive skills. A strength of these models is their emphasis on the analysis of task complexity, a complexity that is independent of whether the task requires verbalized knowing or more implicit procedural problem solving. The increasing articulation and coordination of task components in these models offers a view of how enactive procedures may become more coordinated, articulated, flexible, and inclusive as they are repeatedly applied, without verbal articulation of the procedure itself. Some unique features of enactive procedures for doing things with others are also considered, features that are central to psychoanalytic concerns but that have not been articulated in the literature on cognition.

Finally, nonlinear dynamic systems principles are evoked to account for how the slow transactional process of repeated relational encounters in the psychoanalytic situation can result in increased complexity and organization in the patient's (and analyst's) relational procedures. From a self-organizing systems perspective, this increased articulation destabilizes old forms of organization and eventually crystallizes a shift to an emergent new form of procedural organization that is more complex and coherent.

Part I: Developmental Origins of
Enactive Relational Procedures

Collaborative Dialogue and Coherence in
Enactive Representations

Both the analyst–patient relationship and the parent–infant relationship share a focus on facilitating developmental change—for our purposes here, change particularly in the area of constructing new possibilities for adaptive regulation of intersubjective experiences. In addition, the analyst has the much more demanding charge of facilitating the deconstruction of established but unsatisfying ways of "being with" while simultaneously moving toward the new.

This focus on understanding and deconstructing the old has captured much of the attention of psychoanalytic writers in the past. Psychoanalytic clinicians have inherited a well-articulated descriptive language of individual psychopathology. With this has come an indispensable understanding of how to read some of the intricate and creative defensive maneuvers available to adapt to painful and constricting environments. To some extent, however, psychoanalytic theorists have concentrated on exploring the internalized forms of pathological representations and their emergence in the transference with less attention to articulating the developmental requirements for the co-construction of more flexible, coherent, and adaptive ways of being with others.

Attachment research has demonstrated that the development of coherent "internal working models of attachment" or implicit relational procedures is tied to participation in coherent forms of parent–child dialogue (see van IJzendoorn, 1994, metaanalysis; Main and Goldwyn, 1994). *Dialogue* is being used here in its broadest sense to encompass all avenues of interpersonal communication, including the affective communications inherent in movement, timing of behavior, and speech contour, as well as in gestural and affective signals. *Coherence* is being used as defined in relation to adult attachment representations by Main and Goldwyn (1994), following the philosopher Grice (1975). According to Grice (1975), coherence in communication is achieved by adhering to maxims governing quantity, quality, relation, and manner, that is, being truthful, clear, relevant, and succinct, yet complete. These qualities serve to maximize the overriding communicative principle of cooperation between participants. Thus, coherent dialogue is truthful and collaborative. This definition might also serve as a first-level working model for capturing essential attributes of coherent clinical dialogue as defined in contemporary two-person models.

The attachment research literature offers a perspective on what might be termed some essential features of collaborative dialogue. Studying the early parent–child communication process provides one laboratory for observing how various organizations of dialogue play out over developmental time. Longitudinal attachment studies give some insight into the kinds of parent–child dialogue associated with the child's development of coherent and flexible enactive procedural models for negotiating in relationships. Collaborative and flexible parent–infant dialogues have been termed *open communication* in the developmental attachment literature but this term is subject to misinterpretation. Coherent, or "open," dialogue is characterized, not by parental "openness" in the sense of unmonitored parental self-disclosure, but by parental "openness" to the state of mind of the child, including the entire array of the child's communications, so that particular affective or motive states of the child (anger, passion, distress) are not foreclosed from intersubjective sharing and regulation.

Attachment studies typically assess parental "sensitivity" as the aspect of parental behavior associated with infant attachment security (van IJzendoorn, 1994). However, it became clear in our own work on early interaction that what is required from the parent to merit this description is a continuing attempt to apprehend the infant's current subjective reality (affect state, current desired goal, and level of understanding) and an attempt to devise a response that acknowledges and comments or elaborates on that state ("You want the glass? No, you can't have the glass; it might break. Take this cup." "Maybe this block could be a house. Do you want this to be a house? What kind of house shall we make?") (Lyons-Ruth, Bronfman, and Atwood, 1999; Lyons-Ruth, Bronfman, and Parsons, 1999). Collaborative dialogue, then, is about getting to know another's mind and taking it into account in constructing and regulating interactions. The process of creating adequate intersubjective recognition in development requires close attention to the child's initiatives in interaction because, through these initiatives, the child communicates his or her local and general goals (motives) and their associated meaning structures. Without recognition of one person's initiatives or communications by another, no intersubjectivity or dyadic regulation is possible.

Observation of videotapes of parents and infants during the first year further reveals that the parent actively scaffolds the infant's ability to articulate and communicate his mental states somewhat ahead of the infant's ability to do so himself. Thus, the parent inducts the infant into the role of communicative partner (building on the infant's preadapted ability to participate as a social partner) by responding carefully to infant nonlinguistic initiatives as communications and by taking the infant's turn in conversation until the infant can fill the turn himself, for example, to a 2-month-old: "Does that noise mean you're hungry? Maybe you're hungry. Let's see if you want this water? No? No water? How about juice? Ok, you like that!"

The goodness of fit of the parent's scaffolding activity depends on the parent's ability to develop a sense of the infant's current cognitive capacities, developed likes and dislikes, and store of past experiences. That this knowledge is difficult to attain, approximate at best, fraught with error, and subject to constant revision makes this a challenging process and one easily open to distortion and misattribution by the parent. Another's mind is a terrain that can never be fully known. The difficulty of knowing another's mind guarantees that communication will be fraught with error and require many procedures for disambiguating messages, detecting and correcting misunderstandings, and repairing serious communicative failures, "What's the matter? You don't want your bear? Do you want your blanket? No? Are your new teeth hurting? Maybe you're tired." Thus, empathy should not be viewed as a simple apprehension of one person's state by another but as a complex outcome of a number of skilled communicative procedures for querying and decoding another's subjective reality.

Developmental work, then, has given us systematic access for the first time to the details of collaborative and flexible or incoherent and inflexible verbal and nonverbal interactive processes between parent and child.

Developmental research on attachment relationships has also documented the features of developmental dialogue that are associated with flexibility and resilience in the child's later development. The convergence across studies and across different research traditions is unmistakable. Developmental communication systems that are open to the entire array of affective communications (e.g., Ainsworth et al., 1978); that include both participants' initiatives in a balanced, mutually regulated dialogue (Baldwin, Cole, and Baldwin, 1982); that are characterized by active negotiation and repairing of miscues, misunderstandings, and conflicts of interest (Tronick, 1989; Crockenberg, and Litman, 1990); and that are actively scaffolded by the developmentally more advantaged partner toward more flexible and inclusive forms (e.g., Wood, Bruner, and Ross, 1976) are associated with positive developmental outcomes for the child. These outcomes include affectively positive interpersonal relationships and enactive procedural models for conducting relationships that are coherent, integrated, flexible, and open to new information (see Bretherton, 1988, for a review of this literature).

Based on these emerging studies of communication processes in early development, "coherent communication" in a developmental relationship can be described as having the following features:

1. Active structuring of dialogue around eliciting the child's current and emerging wants, needs, views, likes: Both the importance and the difficulty of knowing another's mind are explicitly acknowledged.
2. Active pursuit of repairs when misunderstanding occurs: Need for mutual contribution to regulation and repair is explicit.
3. Active bridging of dialogue to new levels of awareness by developmentally advantaged partner: Paradox that relationship is mutually regulated in the face of developmental inequality.
4. Active engagement and struggle with the child through transformational periods when awareness of self and others is being reorganized, with attendant recalibration of the extent of the child's initiative and direction of the relationship: Paradox that relationship initiatives are balanced in the face of inequality of power.

Attachment research has further demonstrated that attachment-related encounters in intimate social relationships are regulated by "internal working models" or enactive procedural representations of how to do things with others (van IJzendoorn, 1995, for review). At the adult level, these models are revealed through the verbal discourse of the adult, as research on the Adult Attachment Interview has described (Main, 1993). Because these models are revealed in verbal dialogue, however, does not mean that the models themselves are symbolically represented by the subject, even though they may be symbolically represented by the observing researcher or psychoanalyst. This research has further established that such models can be observed in operation in caregiver–infant transactions, begin to be represented in implicit procedural form early in life, and are mentally reaccessed in new social encounters (see Bretherton, 1988, and Lyons-Ruth, 1991, for reviews). These models also tend to persist into adolescence and adulthood in the absence of major changes in close relationships (see Main, 1993). This work begins to make explicit the partial isomorphism of process and structure, of medium and message, of features of the relational dialogue, and features of the resulting enactive relational procedure.

Attachment research thereby provides general empirical support for the psychoanalytic construct of "internalized objects" while at the same time underscoring the early origins of these models in actual relational transactions. However, "internalization" is occurring at a presymbolic level, prior to the capacity to evoke images or verbal representations of "the object." Thus, the primary form of representation must be one, not of words or images, but one of enactive relational procedures governing "how to do," or what Stern et al. (1998) have called "implicit relational knowing" (see also Lyons-Ruth, 1998).

Enactive Representation and the Implicit Procedural Unconscious

If "objects" are "internalized" from the earliest months of life, not simply as a way of coping with malevolent objects, as Fairbairn (1952) proposed, but as a process of normal development, then a language and a set of constructs are needed to capture how these objects are represented and how such representations change with development. An adequate theory also needs to retain a view of the individually idiosyncratic nature of life experience and the unique elaborations of enactive strategies, internal fantasy, and symbolic meaning that mark the individual. Can cognitive developmental science converge with psychoanalytic thinking to fashion a general theory of the development of enactive relational representation from the earliest months of life?

Both psychoanalytic theory and cognitive science agree that meaning systems include both conscious (e.g., verbalizable or attended to) aspects of experience and unconscious, or implicitly processed, aspects of experience. Implicit processing in modern cognitive science is applied to mental activity that is repetitive and automatic, provides quick categorization and decision making, and operates outside the realm of focal attention and verbalized experience (e.g., Marcel, 1983; Rumelhart and McClelland, 1986; Kihlstrom, 1987). Although not discussed in the cognitive literature, implicit processing may be particularly relevant to the quick and automatic handling of nonverbal affective cues, which are recognized and represented early in infancy in complex social "proto-dialogues" (Trevarthen, 1980), and so have their origins prior to the availability of symbolic communication.

Cognitive–developmental researchers also view thought as involving both conscious and unconscious, or implicit, procedures (Fischer and Pipp, 1984). However, developmental researchers are less quick to equate implicit processing with more repetitive and superficial decision making. For example, Fischer and Pipp (1984) specifically argue against the equation of unconscious processing with the "developmentally primitive" unconscious of Freud, claiming instead that "unconscious thought does not remain static during childhood but demonstrates systematic developments that are structurally parallel to the developments in conscious thought (p. 89)."

The neuropsychology literature approaches the issue of different and parallel forms of mental processing from the study of brain-damaged adults and comes to a converging conclusion. As Schachter and Moscovitch (1984) point out, "The psychological and neurobiological reality of multiple memory systems is ... consistent with a wide range of data from cognitive psychology, neuropsychology, physiological psychology, and we will argue, developmental psychology" (p. 175). They argue for the existence of "at least two distinct and dissociable forms of memory" (p. 174), variously termed procedural versus declarative memory (Cohen and Squire, 1980), "knowing how" versus "knowing that" (Cohen and Squire, 1980), perceptual versus autobiographical memory (Jacoby and Dallas, 1981), "memory in the wide sense" versus "memory in the narrow sense" (Piaget and Inhelder, 1973), or implicit versus explicit memory (Schacter and Buckner, 1998). The implicit form of memory described as "knowing how" refers to the acquisition of skills, maps, and rule-governed adaptive responses that are evident in behavior but remain unconscious, in that they are not represented in symbolic form and are rarely fully translated into language; the explicit form of memory described as "knowing that" involves symbolic or imagistic knowledge that allows facts or experiences to be called into conscious awareness in the absence of the things they stand for. Not surprising to psychoanalysts, the domain of knowledge that is available to conscious awareness through symbolic representation constitutes but a small part of the individual's acquired adaptive knowledge base.

While implicit procedural and explicit declarative forms of knowing interpenetrate one another in normal adult functioning, studies of amnesic adults with a variety of neurological conditions, as well as studies of normal infants, demonstrate the potential dissociability of the two forms of knowledge. For example, amnesics' performances in completing fragmented versions of words benefitted from prior exposure to the word list as much as did normal subjects' performances. However, amnesics' ability to say whether they had seen a specific word before or had even seen the word list before was severely impaired. Implicit procedural knowledge was accrued in the absence of any conscious recall (declarative knowledge) of the learning experience itself. Similar learning effects in the absence of conscious recall occurred on even more complex tasks such as assembling a jigsaw puzzle, learning to apply a complex mathematical rule (the Fibonacci rule), or learning to solve the Tower of Hanoi puzzle (see Schachter and Moscovitch, 1984). Examples cited by Schachter and Moscovitch (1984) that are closer to the concerns of psychoanalysts include a patient of Claparède (1911) who refused to shake Claparède's hand but did not know why she refused. She was not able to recall that the day before she had been pricked with a pin hidden in Claparède's extended hand. In another case, an amnesic was told unusual stories about a series of presented pictures. The next day the patient could not recall that any stories had been told to him. However, he consistently chose titles for the pictures that reflected the unusual themes of those stories.

Cognitive psychologists continue to struggle with numerous issues involved in the more precise specification of these dissociable memory systems (see Anderson, 1982; Schachter and Buckner, 1998). For the purposes of this paper, however, these data make clear that implicit learning, operating outside conscious awareness, is fundamental to complex adult functioning, as well as to infant functioning.

In addition, complex new learning occurs in adulthood through implicit procedural mechanisms, new learning that is not mediated by translation of implicit knowing into symbolic or conscious form, even though words or images may be involved as part of the procedural memory. Particularly relevant to our concerns here, some processes that influence procedural knowing have little effect on declarative memory (such as modality of initial learning), and some processes influencing declarative memory have little effect on implicit learning (such as delay interval after initial learning and level of processing involved in initial learning). Based on all the above data, Schachter and Moscovitch argue for the relative independence of the two memory systems. The implications for our discussion is that change in implicit procedural forms of relational knowing may come about through somewhat different mechanisms than change in conscious declarative forms of knowing.

In recent psychoanalytic writing, the increasing participation of the analyst has been predicated partly on an increasing sense that we gain much more access to these implicit enacted knowings, one's own as well as the patient's, in a more participatory frame. This emerging sense of the implicit procedural unconscious is consistent with modern cognitive research, but its implications for prior models of the unconscious have not yet been explicitly worked out. Such implicit enacted procedures for being with others are central to therapeutic work but are not well captured by previous divisions between primary and secondary process, between ego and id, between verbal and nonverbal, or even by the construct of the dynamic unconscious. Implicit relational procedures are often neither conscious and verbalizable nor repressed in a dynamic sense. They are not reducible to unacceptable drives or impulses and do not have their origins or essence in fantasy. However, implicit relational knowing is likely to be visible in the structure of fantasied interactions, as well as in the enactive structure of real interactions. Seligman (1995) notes that Freud's preconscious may have prefigured this aspect of the unconscious. Stolorow, quoted in Seligman (1995), has advanced the notion of the "pre-reflective unconscious," and Sandler and Sandler (1994) distinguish between the "past unconscious" and the "present unconscious." The Sandlers also offer a careful discussion of Freud's usages of the terms *unconscious* and *preconscious*. An excellent synthesis of the literature on procedural memory from a psychoanalytic viewpoint is also available in Clyman (1991).

Infant research, in particular, has shown us that, long before words are relevant, procedures for being with others are being acquired that vary widely along many dimensions, such as in the likelihood of engaging others in positive exchanges, in the affects that are exhibited or not exhibited to others, in the social and affective information that is elicited from others, or in the effectiveness of procedures for eliciting help or comfort from others. While these procedures develop in adaptation to particular caregiving partners, they are not necessarily equally effective in regulating internal physiological arousal (Spangler and Grossman, 1993; Hertsgaard et al., 1995; Gunnar et al., in press), in protecting exploration and mastery (Cassidy and Berlin, 1994), in adapting to the range of environments encountered in the peer group (Lyons-Ruth, Alpern, and Repacholi, 1993), or in relating to others in adolescence (Kobak and Sceery, 1988). In psychoanalytic work, paying close attention to all transactions in the hour is in keeping with the need to understand the multiple implicit procedural maps of the patient and their breadth, flexibility, and range of application or their discontinuities and inflexibilities. However, if development is not primarily about translating primary process into symbolic form, but about developing implicit adaptive procedures for being with others in a wide range of emotionally charged situations, then making the unconscious conscious does not adequately describe developmental or psychoanalytic change.

Dialogue and Defense

As Ainsworth, Main, and others have further demonstrated, procedural models guiding the early parent–child affective dialogue exhibit various kinds of deletions and distortions or "incoherencies," distortions that analysts have long understood from a one-person, intrapsychic model as defensive (Ainsworth et al., 1978; see Bretherton, 1988, for review). This literature makes clear that implicit two-person processes are integral to the developmental origins of some defenses. This developmental work, tieing nonverbal affective discourse to defensive structure, mirrors the current analytic interest in closely following the process of the two-person dialogue within the hour as it instantiates the deletions and distortions of both participants' implicit relational models.

In the case of less coherent parent–child dialogues, attachment studies have demonstrated that a particular character stance or a particular defensive strategy may constitute one component of a much broader interpersonal arrangement that has endured over a significant period of the patient's life. Thus, some defensive strategies are not best viewed as resulting from a particular intrapsychic conflict or a particular interpersonal perturbation confined to a specific developmental epoch. For example, developmental research has revealed that a child's tendency to suppress vulnerable feelings of anger or distress and to displace attention away from relationships and onto the inanimate world should not be viewed as an obsessional style resulting from control struggles in toddlerhood. Instead, for a sizable number of children (van IJzendoorn, 1994), this stance is reliably evident in the child's behavior by 12 months of age and is related to particular forms of parent–child affective dialogue over the first year of life, including parental suppressed anger and discomfort with close physical contact (Main, Tomasini, and Tolan, 1979) and parental mock surprise expressions to infant anger (Malatesta et al., 1989). These restrictions in parent–child dialogue are further foreshadowed by the parent's style of discourse in attachment-related interviews prior to the child's birth (see van IJzendoorn, 1994, for metaanalytic review).

Even in cases where a traumatic event at a particular developmental period has played a crucial pathogenic role, the continued physiological and intrapsychic effects of traumatic events are related to the quality of parent–child dialogue in relation to the painful event available subsequent to the trauma. For example, recent data tie excessive and sustained reactivity of the stress-responsive hypothalamic-pituitary-adrenal system to impaired collaborativeness in the parent–infant dialogue (Spangler and Grossmann, 1993; Hertsgaard et al., 1995; see Lyons-Ruth and Jacobvitz, 1999, for review). The collaborativeness of the ongoing parent–child dialogue, then, emerges as one potent mediator of whether particular aspects of traumatic experience will be segregated outside the process of ongoing regulation in the parent–child dialogue.

This research literature indicates that implicit two-person processes must be integral to any theory of the development of defenses. However, most theorizing has remained intrapsychically oriented. Attachment theorists have discussed defensive processes as processes that result in the distortion, exclusion, or lack of integration of information or affective experience, with a particular emphasis on the formation and maintenance of multiple inconsistent models of relational experience. From an attachment perspective, Bretherton (1991) cites Stern (1985), Tulving (1972), Craik (1943), and others who point to the potential for multiple models inherent in the representational and memory systems that store human experience.

Other approaches to this issue from both psychoanalytic and attachment theorists stress the role of conflict and intense affect rather than the availability of different modes of mental representation in leading to multiple incompatible models. For example, Main and Hesse (1990), discussing disorganized/disoriented attachment behaviors, stress the role of fear and conflict, in that fear aroused by the attachment figure leads the infant to both activate and inhibit behavioral approaches to the attachment figure when stressed. The simultaneous activation and inhibition postulated stems from the nature of the attachment behavioral system itself, which is normally activated in the presence of fear or threat but which must be simultaneously inhibited in the case where the attachment figure *is* the source of the threat. A similar process is envisioned in adulthood at a representational level, where mental approaches to attachment-related thoughts and feelings may continue to be both activated and inhibited.

Fonagy (1991) advances a somewhat different intrapsychic theory of multiple models derived from clinical object relations theory. In object relations theory, unintegrated models of idealized and devalued versions of self and other have been viewed as based on the defense of splitting, a defense linked to the presence of particularly malevolent representations of important others (Kernberg, 1976). In Fonagy's view, the child's awareness of the malevolence of the caregiver is too painful to tolerate and leads the child to inhibit the ability to reflect on the mental states of self and other, leading to unintegrated and inconsistent representations of central relationships. Fonagy (1991), more explicitly than others, also stresses the lowered developmental level of the resulting mental representations.

A more radical and social constructivist view of the defenses, including splitting, is inherent in recent attachment research, however. Attachment researchers have demonstrated more dramatically than any other group the interactive basis for the deletions and distortions prominent in many implicit relational strategies. If negative affects, particularly hateful ones, produce hostile attack, intense devaluation, shaming, or withdrawal by the parent, they may be excluded from further discourse. Exclusion of negative affects from interaction also excludes these affects from the integrated developmental elaboration and understanding of anger-related behaviors, affects, and experiences that might come from more balanced acceptance and inclusion in interaction and discussion.

Attachment research has consistently grounded defensive maneuvers in infancy, such as infant avoidance, in the behavioral and affective responses of the caregivers, responses based on their own implicit models of relationships. These interpersonal defensive maneuvers have been viewed as interactive and adaptive in origin rather than purely intrapsychic in origin. Recent research on infants with disorganized attachment behavior has also tied these conflicted forms of infant behavior to fearful and hesitant or hostile and frightening responses of the caregiver (see Lyons-Ruth, Bronfman and Atwood, 1999; Lyons-Ruth, Bronfman, and Parsons, 1999). These disorganized attachment behaviors in infancy also predict later forms of role-reversal with the parent during the preschool years (Main, Kaplan, and Cassidy, 1985). These findings point to the parent's difficulty in attending to and balancing the initiatives of the infant with those of the self, with the ensuing collapse of intersubjective space so that only one party's subjective reality is acknowledged. This collapse of intersubjective space in the interactions between parent and child may also lead to the impaired capacity of borderline patients to integrate conflicting representations and to mentally reflect on the subjective states of self and other, as noted by Fonagy (1991).

This view of defenses as partially grounded in the structure of exchanges with important others is also congruent with the increasing awareness among analysts that interactions between patient and analyst instantiate the defensive exclusions or contradictions of the patient's implicit procedural knowledge. Currently, mutual reflection on "enactments" in the therapy is seen as a rich source of insight about these implicit procedural knowings, including the resort to defensive distortion or exclusion of information. Developmental research further establishes that many of the defensive deletions and distortions evident in enactments have "two-person" origins.

Part II: Enactive Relational Representation and the Process of Change

Because changes in the organization of meaning systems are what we are generally referring to when we talk about both developmental change and psychoanalytic change, accounting for changes in meaning systems is critical to both developmental and psychoanalytic theory. For developmental theory, in particular, change cannot be adequately described as simply making the unconscious conscious. Instead, new ways of being with others are being acquired. Yet no literature has grappled extensively with how "working models," "internalized objects," or "implicit procedural meanings" become either more articulated and complex over developmental time or reworked during psychoanalytic treatment. A sufficiently powerful model of change in implicit relational knowing is likely to require the synthesis of insights from both developmental science and psychoanalytic theory.

A Control Systems Model of Mind

What does current cognitive–developmental science have to offer a psychoanalytic theory of meaning? Findings from 30 years of cognitive–developmental research are converging with similar results from the neurosciences and from studies of adult cognition to yield the following general insights into the construction of meaning systems, insights that are also congenial to the clinical experience of mind and meaning.

1. The mind is naturally fractionated, with meaning systems often unintegrated with one another (e.g., Fischer and Granott, 1995).
2. Mental processing occurs at several levels in parallel, as well as in sequence (Marcel, 1983; Fischer and Granott, 1995).
3. All adapted activity expresses mental structure (Fischer, 1980).

4. All cognition is essentially re-cognition in that new learning automatically reorganizes old learning to some extent (Edelman, 1987; Freeman, 1990).
5. Meanings are co-constructed in interaction with the minds and artifacts of a particular culture (Vygotsky, 1962; Bruner, Olver, and Greenfield, 1966).
6. In domains of meaning with rich cultural investment (the provision of many minds and artifacts to assist in the mental articulation of a domain), meaning systems will develop through higher levels of organization, that is, will become articulated and integrated into higher-order coordinations and proceduralized to allow more elements into working memory more rapidly and completely than in domains without support (Bruner, Olver, and Greenfield, 1966; Fischer, 1980; Anderson, 1982).
7. Developmentally, constraints of working memory and processing speed set an upper limit on the level of organization in adaptive action that can be achieved, but up to this upper limit, level of organization realized will vary widely across domains, depending on the degree of support for elaborating the representational domain (Case, 1991; Fischer, 1980).
8. Even if an optimal level of complexity of thought can be demonstrated in a given domain, use of that optimal level may still vary widely with context (Fischer and Granott, 1995).

If these general features of thought are applied to implicit working models of relationships, we would expect to find that the flexible and integrated organization of implicit relational experience is particularly dependent on the quality and extent of participation by a relational partner. This dependence on the quality of the partner's participation also implies that implicit relational knowing is particularly vulnerable to fractionation and lack of integration among the implicit meaning systems governing relational behavior. That is, lack of mental integration may occur not only because of intrapsychic defensive processes, but also because of the absence of collaborative relationships within which to articulate and integrate relational understanding and ways of being. Areas of potentially conflicting enactive knowledge may remain unintegrated with one another, as occurs in splitting, and in addition, potentially conflicting symbolic and enactive knowings may operate in parallel without integration across modes of representation.

Recent cognitive–developmental theory (Fischer, 1980; Case, 1991; Fischer and Granott, 1995) offers the most powerful current model for how meaning systems and their associated adaptive skills for doing things in the world change with development. Modern cognitive–developmental theory sees development as involving the construction of progressively more complex control (or meaning) systems. These control systems are properties of both the person and the environmental context in which they develop. Cognition, action, and emotion are all interrelated products of these control systems. The best current description of how an enactive control system changes emphasizes the gradual microprocess by which single developed skills, or enactive relational procedures, are coordinated with other single skills or procedures to form second-level coordinated thought structures, which are, in turn, coordinated with one another. For each procedure one must learn to achieve a particular outcome reliably over a set of environmental variations and then coordinate that procedure with a related procedure. For example, after a conflict with his mother, a 2-year-old might learn to calm his distress from a variety of intensity levels, using a variety of supports (thumb, blanket, parental hug, shift of attention) and then coordinate this enactive procedure with a second set of procedures for engaging in playful games with the parent, leading to a set of coordinated second-level control structures for "making up," for moving from distress in relation to the parent to a calm state and ultimately back to positive engagement and play. This enactive relational procedure might then be coordinated with procedures for interacting with playmates rather than parents, so that a coordinated procedural control system develops for making up with playmates after a conflict.

It is important to note that, although words are used for the first time in the service of enactive relational procedures during toddlerhood, the embedding of words into procedures does not make the organization of the procedure itself available to reflective thought or verbal representation. The 3-year old may be able to verbalize meanings of "good" and "bad," but he cannot represent consciously or verbally that he inhibits his impulse to reach out for comfort to his father because his father's physical withdrawal and cold voicetone communicate disapproval of comfort-seeking. The organizational structure of most relational behavior remains unconscious and implicit even though the child's new words and understandings may be incorporated into these implicit procedures.

Fischer (1980) and Case (1991) both detail this developmental process of gradual coordination of more complex, integrated, and inclusive implicit procedures or control structures through a series of developmental levels. The reader should consult Fischer (1980) and Case (1991) for their detailed expositions of how particular domains of procedural knowing are assembled component by component, during the years from infancy to adulthood. These theories have extended the older Piagetian framework in a number of ways that deemphasize his monolithic and hierarchical stage structures, replacing them with a set of more varied and context-responsive "skills" or modular meaning systems. These modular meaning systems require environmental support but operate within the general constraints of memory capacity and processing speed available at a given age.

In contrast to older views, there is no simple uniform progression through a series of stages, and people do not operate at a particular level across tasks. The series of levels and sublevels outlined by Fischer (1980) or Case (1991) represent, not epochs of development, but an analysis of task complexity, of the level of implicit mental articulation needed to accomplish a set of adaptive actions. The level of complexity of a given child's or adult's control systems typically varies widely across tasks. Development is viewed as a process of developing concurrently along a number of pathways that may be only loosely or not at all coordinated by level of articulation achieved. Even along a given pathway, level of complexity of thought and action will vary with contextual factors from day to day. To quote Fischer, "People do not have integrated, fundamentally logical minds. Instead, we have many control systems that are naturally separate, although potentially we can develop coordination and integration of many of them" (p. 153). This view is clearly consistent with clinical experience, in that an individual's relational repertoire for doing things with others may be quite discrepant from the person's skills in other areas.

These emerging context-sensitive and modular views of the development of meaning are congenial to many of the clinical insights of psychoanalysis. They emphasize the integral relations between meaning systems and adapted behavior; the fractionated and context-specific nature of both symbolic and procedural meaning systems, the importance of cultural partners in scaffolding or co-constructing representational systems to more flexible and inclusive forms; and the gradual, iterative, yet individually idiosyncratic process through which meaning systems become more articulated, integrated, and inclusive. More specifically than in the attachment literature, these researchers delineate the processing constraints on the elaboration of both procedural and symbolic meaning systems during particular developmental periods and delineate the gradual process through which components of a task or meaning domain are differentiated and systematically coordinated into more flexible and inclusive systems.

Although the language of cognitive science is often uncongenial to clinicians, a model of the slow articulation of a domain of meaning within a set of developmental constraints is likely to describe aspects of the construction of implicit and explicit relational knowing both during development and during psychoanalytic therapy. Contemporary neuroscience also describes mental organization as proceeding through a gradually accruing complexity of neuronal connections until a critical point is reached where higher level organization emerges spontaneously (Edelman, 1987). The neuroscience literature also stresses the individually idiosyncratic nature of the accruing neuronal organizations but the seemingly paradoxical convergence of these idiosyncratic pathways on species-typical behavioral outcomes. Somehow developmentally, we tend to arrive at a similar place through vastly different routes. These models of the increasing articulation and organization of both neuronal systems and relational procedures potentially provide support for a meaning-focused psychoanalytic enterprise from contemporary scientific views and create fertile ground for more collaborative dialogue across psychoanalytic and developmental disciplines.

Parallel Mental Processing

Recent awareness of the parallel nature of much cognitive activity and the sharp constraints on what can ever be the subject of sustained focal (conscious) attention has led to a more general realization that thinking progresses to highly complex, formal modes through the development of enactive procedures that are not easily, and never completely, translated into a verbal, explicitly retrievable medium (e.g., Fischer and Granott, 1995; Marcel, 1983). This enactive dimension is most obvious in the domains that do not easily lend themselves to verbal expression, such as musical composition or performance, complex artistic or athletic skills, and spatial or architectural expertise. However, the increased complexity of implicit knowing that comes with repeated exposure or repeated doing is also intrinsic to the most symbol-laden domains as well, such as the writing of scientific papers or the analysis of literature.

Knowing how to proceed in intimate relationships may be another domain in which complex knowledge is constructed outside a predominantly verbal medium, in which procedures for skilled interaction, incorporating a range of subtle affective cues, develop through a series of more articulated and integrated coordinations largely outside the domain of verbalized knowledge and conscious awareness. Clearly, as a species, we still have a very sparse systematic verbalized knowledge base for understanding how human interaction "works," even though we enact it daily at highly skilled levels. Even in the analytic literature, there is often a large gap between insights systematized in the literature and the subtlety and complexity of what the analyst implicitly knows and does clinically. Implicit clinical knowing, then, also proceeds to high levels of complexity outside the medium of words, even though systematized, verbalized knowledge is highly valued in the field.

In order to emphasize that the structure of thinking is inherent in action, Fischer (1980) calls his cognitive–developmental theory a theory of skill development. In his view, cognition at every level is fundamentally about learning to control a range of actions, whether physical or mental actions, in the service of achieving a particular outcome in the world, over a specific set of variations in environmental input. For example, at the sensorimotor level, between 9 and 12 months, the infant learns how to coordinate his focus of attention with the caregiver's, by using a variety of vocal sounds and gestures to redirect her focus of attention to coincide with his, no matter what her physical position or current focus of attention may be (see Bretherton, McNew, and Beeghly-Smith, 1981). A related, but much more complex, skill at the abstract level of thinking is to coordinate one's parenting and career identities over time with the parenting and career identities of one's spouse through joint negotiation and decision making (see Fischer, 1980). These examples point to the mentally organized structure of behaviors that are also imbued with strong affects serving basic survival needs. Both the cognitive–developmental and attachment research literatures, then, converge on the notion that implicit relational knowing is one realm where organized enactive or implicit procedural knowledge develops from the first months of life largely outside the arena of symbolic or verbalized knowledge.

Melvin Lewis (1995), in a related argument regarding amnesia and transference, also discusses the distinction between procedural and declarative memory and proposes a developmental shift hypothesis to account for infantile amnesia. According to his hypothesis, some early developmental structures, such as primary process and sensorimotor thought, are maintained as they are throughout development and would be manifested in preverbal, affective, sensory, and motoric memory patterns. In contrast, later memory functions, especially those involving language, would change extensively with development. He speculates that the concept of infantile amnesia as a result of repression may not be viable since nonverbal forms of memory can be recovered from infancy onward. He concludes, "The apparent lack of verbal access might have nothing at all to do with repression; it might simply be that early memories are encoded in a prelanguage form and that we have been looking for the wrong representation of very early memories—for words rather than for physiological responses, behavior and affect" (p. 410).

While his argument converges with the view advanced here that implicit relational representations are constructed from the first months of life, the model advanced here differs from this implied "developmental shift" view. In a developmental shift view, affective and behavioral representational systems that do not become more complex with development are contrasted with verbal systems that emerge during the second year and that *do* become more complex. A more powerful and general model is a parallel systems model, rather than a developmental shift model. In a parallel systems model, the affective and behavioral representations guiding interactions with others continue to become more articulated and complex with development, with newly acquired verbal capacity incorporated into interactive strategies, but the strategies themselves not dependent on verbal articulation. This is clearly in keeping with the complexity of the transference phenomena that present clinically. In this view, affective and behavioral representations are not *pre*verbal; they are simply not primarily verbal.

Following Bretherton (1991), Stern (1995), and others, these implicit relational procedures can be described as organized around a variety of local and superordinate goals and as including both interactive procedures and their associated webs of cognitive and affective meanings. These multivalent relational schemes would include not only verbal or verbalizable "cognitive" meanings if these are available, but also a rich web of imagistic "fantasies" and affect-related physiological sensations and the implicit relational knowing of how these meanings and fantasies are related to social actions. The integral connections between cognition and "valuation," or feeling, which is required in this model, have also been emphasized by Damascio (1994) and Edelman (1987) on the basis of recent neuroscience research. Stern (1995) has also recently delineated the multidimensional nature of early relational schemes as experienced in parent–infant psychotherapy.

If representations of "how to do things with others" integrate semantic and affective meaning with behavioral/interactive procedures, then a particular implicit relational procedure may be accessed through multiple routes, and representational change may be set in motion by changes in affective experience, cognitive understanding, or interactive encounters, without necessarily assigning privileged status to a particular dimension, such as interpretation. Stern (1995) has made a related point in relation to parent–infant psychotherapy, where the therapist's intervention may be targeted toward the parent's representation of her own experience, at the therapist–parent transference relationship, or at the parent–infant interaction itself. Mobilizing change across more aspects of these multidimensional thinking, feeling, and doing schemes at once will presumably enhance the effectiveness of the change process, assuming appropriate pace and timing so as not to overload the patient.

Task Structure in the Relational Domain:
A Common Element in Developmental and Psychoanalytic Change

With the increasing influence of infant research, psychoanalytic theorists have struggled with the extent to which the parent–infant or parent–child dyad provides a useful analogy to the therapeutic dyad (e.g., Mitchell, 1988; Wolff, 1996). Following the work of Fischer and Case, I would propose that an essential common structuring element in developmental and psychoanalytic change is the task structure intrinsic to the process of getting to know another's mind. Both developmental and psychoanalytic change in how one conducts oneself in intimate relationships must be constrained by the series of differentiations and integrations required for the construction of collaborative procedures for acting in relationships. The continuing developmental construction of higher-order coordinations of mental entities that Case and Fischer have described in abstract terms have been systematically studied in relation to the child's progressively more complex ability to conceptualize the activity of other minds (see Hobson, 1993; Selman, 1980). The literature on the child's emerging "theory of mind" documents the child's evolving ability to think about thinking, including his own thinking. Self-reflective function, which Fonagy (1991) in particular has highlighted, is closely related to, but generally lags developmentally behind, reflection on the other's subjectivity (Landry and Lyons-Ruth, 1980).

Psychoanalytic discussions of representation usually involve the representation of subjective states, so the developmental emergence of a number of successive levels of "thinking about thinking" introduces a number of potential levels of "representation" of intersubjective events. Intersubjective awareness, then, is not best discussed in terms of whether conscious awareness or symbolic representation has been achieved per se. Instead, we must consider what level of "thinking about thinking" has been fluently achieved and procedurally integrated over which types of affective and relational contexts. Whether starting in early childhood or in adulthood, one must first elaborate an awareness of how one's own mental life is both similar to and different from that of others to elaborate further an understanding of how to make those similarities and differences explicit in dialogue and then to construct procedures for negotiating with the other in the face of differences. The same series of understandings must be elaborated by the developing child.

The essential features of both the verbal and the implicit procedural meaning systems constituting the domain of relational knowing are still poorly described and understood in both the developmental, cognitive, and psychoanalytic literatures. Developmental work on the child's emerging theory of mind (e.g., Carpenter, Nagell, and Tomasello, 1998; Hobson, 1993), work on the relational deficits characterizing autistic individuals (e.g., Hobson, 1993), and research on children's social understanding (Selman, 1980) contribute some detail from the research literature. The rich body of psychoanalytic descriptive work on severe character disorders also offers the potential for a theory of how the domain of intersubjective knowing is elaborated or remains unelaborated, under normal and abnormal conditions (e.g., Fonagy, 1991). This body of work first needs to be freed of prior untenable developmental assumptions, however (e.g., Westen, 1990; Lyons-Ruth, 1991).

Psychoanalytic work on the organization of the intersubjective worlds of child and adult patients and developmental research on the construction of intersubjective understanding are complementary lenses refracting a common underlying domain of knowing. In the "common structure" view offered here, the parent–child relationship is not a metaphor for the adult–patient relationship or vice-versa. Instead, both offer unique, but converging, routes to describing how human beings coconstruct a set of procedures and understandings for negotiating the intersubjective field. Understanding how mind constructs the intersubjective field, whether during childhood or adulthood, is crucial to the further development of both psychoanalysis and developmental science. In this view both developmental and psychoanalytic change emerge from the dynamic interplay of the multiple constraints of intersubjective task structure, working memory capacity, and the quality and extent of participation of interacting partners. This complex constructivist view allows us to move away from a monolithic view of developmental sequence. It also allows us to see similarities in the processes of developmental and psychoanalytic change, not in terms of the adult's regression to or fixation at a stage of infancy or childhood, but in terms of the similarities through which humans of all ages approach and progress through the mastering of the complex task domain of negotiating with other minds.

Unique Features of Relational Control Systems

Analytic thinkers and infant researchers would both call for several additions to these cognitive models of meaning construction, however. Both analytic theorists and infancy researchers would call attention to the special problems presented by the need to know and be known by another mind, a condition that is a prerequisite for the construction of meaning systems regarding how to be with others. The elaboration of notions of intersubjectivity, or how two minds interface with one another, is an intrinsically collaborative process that depends on one mind becoming reasonably well known to at least one other mind. This necessary extended intersubjective collaboration can create unique and idiosyncratic contexts in which interpersonal meaning systems are elaborated, unlike the regularities and multiple examples more characteristic of commerce with the physical world. The availability of a learning context for elaborating intersubjective meanings is then highly constrained by the frequency and particular quality of the partner's participation in what Tronick (1998) has referred to as "the dyadic expansion of consciousness" (see also Sander, 1995).

Psychoanalytic thinkers in particular would also call attention to the powerful motive systems and accompanying strong affects that impact the elaboration of intersubjective meanings more strongly than they impact the elaboration of concepts of the physical world. The segregation of meanings associated with powerful negative affects has been a central insight of psychoanalytic observation since its inception. To date, cognitive researchers have not attempted to develop a thorough analysis of the meaning systems that guide intimate relationships. The cognitive term *sensorimotor intelligence* itself fails to acknowledge the existence early in infancy of an affective communication system served by an elaborate expressive facial musculature that is unique to the human species (Izard, 1978). In addition to the increasingly complex sensorimotor coordinations that are assembled over the first 2 years, there are also increasingly complex affective and interpersonal coordinations that are co-constructed, as delineated particularly in the attachment literature, as well as in related studies by Tronick, Sander, and Stern. These increasingly complex coordinations of interpersonal action and intersubjective awareness are likely to follow the microdevelopmental steps in the articulation of meaning systems explicated by Fischer and Case. That the first extended tutorial in intersubjective awareness is usually conducted with an attachment figure whose presence and participation are necessary for the child's survival further imbues these exchanges with powerful affects. How these affect systems organize, fragment, or distort the development of meaning systems has not been considered in any depth in the cognitive literature (but see Damasio, 1994).

Affective features, as well as cognitive features, are likely to be central to psychopathology, however. The *complexity* of one's verbal reasoning about others, and perhaps of one's implicit procedural knowing, has no simple relation to psychopathology. Verbal reasoning about others can be highly developed in the context of severe character issues and maladaptive behaviors (see work by Selman, 1980). Therapeutic work seems to be about identifying ways of proceeding, or assumptions about others, that are maladaptive outside the initial context of learning but may or may not be less complex. Instead, they may be more imbued with rage or fear, less integrated with other procedural knowings, less effective in modulating internal physiological stress responses, or more likely to involve fearful or hostile interpretations of others' behavior. Deconstructing complex, but maladaptive, ways of being with, while simultaneously co-constructing more adaptive but equally complex new ways of being together, is likely to involve a slow mutual journey through a series of intersubjective encounters that catalyze the construction of new control systems. A model that integrates motivational and affective processes with the increasing articulation and organization of relational control structures seems necessary.

Viewed developmentally, the domain of implicit relational knowing becomes more complex over normal development, largely through apprentice learning and participant observation rather than verbal instruction. Whether the gradual process of differentiation and coordination of components of meaning (or action) described in the developmental literature will prove useful to understanding the developmental construction or therapeutic reconstruction of implicit relational knowing remains to be fully explored. However, the question of how the meaning systems comprising the domain of implicit relational knowing develop and change needs to be grappled with by both developmental and psychoanalytic theorists.

Conflict, Negative Affect, and Fragmented or Dissociated Enactive Procedures

Procedural models for being with others are organized at first according to the developmental level of understanding available at the time they are taking form and may or may not become reorganized over time in accord with later levels of understanding. So an implicit relational procedure, along with its associated meanings and values, may remain at the initial level of representation or may be only partially updated from time to time, leaving coexisting variations at succeeding developmental levels (probably the norm for most areas of experience), or may have been repeatedly reaccessed and in the process reconstructed over time so that developmentally earlier versions have been largely replaced (see Edelman, 1987). Many such implicit procedures for how to negotiate affectively charged exchanges with others are a part of what is being brought to the psychoanalyst.

From the perspective of normal development, lack of articulation and integration of either implicit or explicit representational systems can have many origins, including developmental limitations in meaning-making at a particular age, implicit rules of family engagement that exclude particular ways of relating, implicit rules that include procedural action but refuse verbal acknowledgment, traumatic experiences whose implications threaten other survival-necessary "ways of being with," and the usual disjunctions of human life where somewhat contradictory implicit procedures may evolve governing, for example, public versus private life, sibling versus peer relations, or same-sex versus opposite-sex interactions.

Conflict at the level of implicit procedural representation inheres in the tension between the goals and needs of the child and the responses of the varied caregiving environments that are encountered developmentally. While other forms of discontinuity or limitation in procedures may exist, the ones most relevant to psychoanalytic theory are those associated with imbalanced interpersonal interaction, need frustration, and negative affect. Inadequate response to central goals and needs of the child creates both negative affects and areas of exchange that become foreclosed to further negotiation, articulation, and integration. Thus, disruptions or imbalances in interpersonal transactions are initially isomorphic with discontinuities or inadequacies in relational procedures and are associated with experienced conflict around the frustration of central goals. Conflict among the child's competing goals per se (such as to preserve a good relationship with the parent or to insist on one's own way; to do away with father or to love father) are unlikely to result in lasting difficulties in and of themselves unless corresponding conflicts between the goals of parent and child interfere with their developmental resolution (Fischer and Watson, 1981).

When flexible mental and emotional access to most levels of experience has been available within a development-enhancing dialogue, the resulting relational control systems will be reasonably well integrated, with both interpersonally contested issues and internally contradictory goals and meanings struggled with and resolved *to the extent necessary* to negotiate the world. If many of the patient's goals have been overridden and excluded from further interaction, negative affects related to the frustration of those goals will remain unresolved while caregiver negative affects toward the pursuit of those goals will also be represented. These points of unresolved conflict become internalized as discontinuities in implicit procedures, discontinuities often marked by strong conflicting emotions. Likewise, if relational goals have been enacted in relationships in forms that conflict with what is acknowledged or have been enacted in contradictory forms whose contradictions are never confronted, the resulting implicit procedural representations will be segregated, fragmented, or contradictory, with little opportunity to update, articulate, and integrate implicit "ways of being with" as new developmental capacities become available (see Bretherton, 1988). Therapeutic work will then be occurring around the fault lines where interactive negotiations have failed, goals remain aborted, negative affects are unresolved, conflict is experienced, and implicit procedural representations have become segregated from one another.

Viewing "internalized objects" or "transferences" as relational control systems governed by implicit procedural models makes clearer that segregated or fragmented implicit procedural maps will not only be imbued with conflicted affects but are likely to be underdeveloped in various ways compared to procedures that have developed in relationships characterized by more coherent communication. Alternately, one can view procedures developed under conditions of more restricted communication, not as "underdeveloped," but as differently developed under conditions where barriers to self-expression and the associated segregation and fragmentation of relational control procedures are valued and enforced.

Removing affective barriers to new ways of being with others is only one aspect of the change process, however; new procedures that are more articulated, integrated, and adapted to current reality must be developed. In traditional theory, the work after initial "insight" is achieved has proceeded under the rubric of "working through." If relational knowing is as much implicit and procedural as symbolic, the work of elaborating new implicit procedures for being with others must occur at enactive as well as symbolic levels.

A final subtle shift occurs in adopting a representational systems model of mind in that we must struggle with the issue of creating new representational structures. If representational systems are always in a process of reconstruction with every activation (see Edelman, 1987; Freeman, 1990), then analytic work is always involved in the creation of the new and the reworking of the old simultaneously. While "making the unconscious conscious" or verbalized may be one part of this co-constructive process, developmental research, in particular, suggests that the emergence of new implicit relational procedures developmentally is not simply about putting unconscious motivations or implicit procedures into words, but about new forms of organization emerging as new forms of "being with" are scaffolded between parent and child.

Nonlinear Models of Change: Increasing
Elaboration and Emergent Properties

Analytic theory and practice have always recognized both the slow, incremental processes of forming an alliance and working through, as well as the observed major shifts in organization presumed to be attendant on a successful interpretation. Edelman's (1987) theory of neuronal group selection also points to the importance both of the small incremental processes by which certain neuronal groups gain articulation at the expense of other potential pathways and of the relatively sudden emergence of a higher-order organization once the number of reciprocal and recursive feedback loops reaches a critical point. Dynamic systems theory also draws our attention to the sudden emergence of new forms of organization with increased articulation of the constituents of the system (Thelen and Smith, 1994). Edelman's theory of neuronal groups further indicates that the small elaborations that occur as a neuronal group is slowly constructed or reconstructed with use *are* the engine of change, with a higher-order organization emerging as a function of the critical mass of new and overlapping articulated elements attained.

Applying the lens of these theories of self-organizing biological systems, what may need more emphasis is the extended period of intersubjective encounters between patient and analyst that have increased the complexity and organization of some aspects of the intersubjective field at the expense of others. This idiosyncratic and slow process of elaborating some aspects of neuronal organization at the expense of others—or, at another level of analysis, of slowly creating new implicit relational procedures—is the work that creates competing and destabilizing mental and behavioral structures. Viewed from a self-organizing systems perspective, as increasingly articulated competing organization emerges, the old organization is destabilized, with an increasing subjective sense of creative disorder and internal flux (Thelen and Smith, 1994; see also Stolorow, in press). At this point of increasing instability, the analyst (and the patient as well) may be able to crystallize the shift in mental organization and awareness to a new, and often more complex, form by making the additional re-cognitions needed through interpretation. Once this state of instability and flux is achieved, however, the reorganizing re-cognitions might also come about through an emotionally salient series of transactions with the analyst, as loosely captured by the term *corrective emotional experience,* or through a powerful transaction between the two participants when the analyst is forced somewhat out of role, as described under the rubric of enactment. The more distal source of change, however, is not the proximal crystallizing encounter or interpretation but the preceding long period of destabilizing patient–analyst encounters.

Such a model seems to capture well the feel of clinical work and is foreshadowed in much of previous analytic writing regarding the need to prepare for the interpretation. In the older literature, however, the focus was on elaborating the patient's symbolic representations via clarification and interpretation. The newer developmental and neuroscience literatures suggest that, in addition to conscious symbolic elaboration, patient and analyst must be working simultaneously at an implicit relational level to create increasingly collaborative forms of dialogue. Developmental research suggests that collaborative dialogue includes careful attention to the particular state of the other's intersubjective experience, open acceptance of a broad range of affects, active scaffolding to more inclusive levels of dialogue, and engaged struggle and intersubjective negotiation through periods when the other's mind is changing and new ways of relating are needed. Coherence of mind and perfectly collaborative communication are abstractions that will never be realized given the many simultaneous levels of human communication, the natural fractionation of representational systems, the constant process of new relational encounters, and the powerful affects that resist certain kinds of exchanges or insights. However, in developmental attachment studies, more inclusive, succinct, noncontradictory, and truthful forms of parent–child dialogue have been shown to yield more coherent internal working models of attachment and more flexible, integrated, and adaptive implicit relational procedures and to confer developmental advantages in "average, expectable" environments.

A corollary of this view of developmental process is that development is never "arrested" but takes different forms with different relational experiences. Thus, we must understand both the implicit and explicit relational meaning systems that *did* develop *and* the enactive relational procedures that *might have* developed under other circumstances and might serve the child or adult better in her current context. Patient and therapist are inevitably working simultaneously at affective, cognitive, and enactive levels to deconstruct the old, more limited, or more negatively toned procedures or meanings, while simultaneously constructing more integrated, flexible, and hopeful ways of making meaning and being together.

In the process of normal development, implicit relational procedures are continually being modified through new forms of dialogue that are more collaborative and inclusive, forms that achieve more specific recognition of the other's subjectivity and that allow the elaboration of new expressions of agency and affect. For an adult patient, more collaborative and inclusive dialogue may involve partially translating previously implicit procedural knowing into words, while for the young child the work may operate entirely at the implicit level through interactive play that is largely noninterpretation-based (see Ablon, 1996). For example, the therapist might engage with the child's fear of aggressive interactions by permissive and assertive moves in collaborative play that are never raised to the level of interpretation. The degree of verbalized self-awareness that is useful would depend on the usual level of verbalized self-reflective function characteristic of a child of a given age. In this conception any sharp distinction between insight-promotion and "corrective experience" or "developmental help" is not primary as long as there is a psychoanalytically informed engagement around the organization of the child's or adult's implicit and explicit relational meaning systems.

This conception of therapeutic process as the simultaneous deconstruction of maladaptive control structures and the increasing articulation of competing control structures offers a more general conceptualization of the several levels of process that are coming together in a new emerging organization at a moment of therapeutic change. If representational change involves not only cognition or "insight" but also changes in affectively rich "ways of being with," a shift in organization must also involve a reorganization of the analyst's and patient's ways of being together. Therefore, moments of reorganization must involve a new kind of intersubjective meeting that occurs in a new "opening" in the interpersonal space, allowing both participants to become agents toward one another in a new way. This "opening" between the two, which in this conception is part of a state of destabilization and flux created by an emergent new organization, allows new initiatives and spontaneous interpersonal actions to be applied toward constructing a new or different intersubjective arrangement (and representation). This new organization is not simply a product of the individual patient's intrapsychic work, however, but of the working out of new relational possibilities with the analyst. The analyst's specific participation as a new kind of relational partner is part of the "something more" that allows an integrated affective and relational change, in concert with the conscious insight that may or may not accompany the emergence of the new order. A more elaborated statement of this view of change in analytically oriented treatment is articulated in Stern et al. (1998).

Conclusions

A conceptual framework for understanding psychoanalytic and developmental change in implicit relational knowing is offered that is congruent with current developmental and neuroscientific research and congenial to the clinical "feel" of extended analytically oriented treatment. Three major shifts from previous analytic theory seem necessary to accommodate new research. First, developmental work makes clear that characteristics of the two-person dialogue make central contributions to the form of "internalized objects" or implicit relational procedures that are constructed by the child, as well as to the defensive deletions and distortions that mark those implicit procedures. Second, a theory of implicit or enacted procedural meaning is needed that is not isomorphic with previous conceptions of the dynamic unconscious. Third, a conception of how procedures for being with others become more articulated, adapted, and inclusive is needed that does not rely solely or primarily on translating procedural knowing into symbolic form. In summary, the analytically central concepts of motivation, affect, conflict, and defense need to be integrated with a theory of the development of implicit relational knowing to account more fully for both clinical and developmental phenomena.

REFERENCES

Ablon, S. (1996), The therapeutic action of play. *J. Amer. Acad. Child & Adoles. Psychiat.*, 35:545–547.
Ainsworth, M. D. S., Blehar, M., Waters, E. & Wall, S. (1978), *Patterns of Attachment.* Hillsdale, NJ: Lawrence Erlbaum.
Anderson, J. (1982), Acquisition of cognitive skill. *Psycholog. Rev.*, 89:369–406.

Baldwin, A., Cole, R. & Baldwin, C. (1982), Parental pathology, family interaction, and the competence of the child in school. *Monogr. Soc. Res. Child Develop.,* 47:197.

Beebe, B. & Lachman, F. M. (1994), Representation and internalization in infancy: Three principles of salience. *Psychoanal. Psychol.,* 11:127–165.

Bollas, C. (1987), *The Shadow of the Object.* London: Free Association Books.

Boston Process of Change Study Group (1998), Interventions that effect change in psychotherapy: A model based on infant research. *Infant Mental Health J.,* 19:277–353.

Bowlby, J. (1969), *Attachment and Loss: Vol. 1. Attachment.* New York: Basic Books.

Bretherton, I. (1988), Open communication and internal working models: Their role in the development of attachment relationships. In: *Nebraska Symposium on Motivation: Socio-emotional Development,* ed. R. A. Thompson. Lincoln, NE: University of Nebraska Press, (pp. 57–113).

———— (1991), Pouring new wine into old bottles: The social self as internal working model. In: *Minnesota Symposia on Child Development: Vol. 23. Self Process and Development,* ed. M. R. Gunnar & L. A. Sroufe. Hillsdale, NJ: Lawrence Erlbaum, pp. 1–41.

———— McNew, S. & Beeghly-Smith, M. (1981), Early person knowledge as expressed in verbal and gestural communications: When do infants acquire a "theory of mind"? In: *Infant Social Cognition,* ed. M. E. Lamb & L. R. Sherrod. Hillsdale, NJ: Lawrence Erlbaum, pp. 333–373.

Bruner, J. S., Olver, R. R. & Greenfield, P. M. (1966), *Studies in Cognitive Growth.* New York: Wiley.

Carpenter, M., Nagell, K. & Tomasello, M. (1998), Social cognition, joint attention, and communicative competence from 9 to 15 months of age. *Monogr. Soc. Research Child Develop.,* 63:1–174.

Case, R. (1991), *The Mind's Staircase.* Hillsdale, NJ: Lawrence Erlbaum.

Cassidy, J. & Berlin, L. J. (1994), The insecure/ambivalent pattern of attachment: Theory and research. *Child Develop.,* 65:971–991.

Claparède, E. (1911), Reconnaissance et moitié. (Recognition and me-ness.) *Arch. Psychol.,* 11:79–90. In: *Organization and Pathology of Thought,* ed. D. Rapaport. New York: Columbia University Press, 1951.

Clyman, R. (1991), The procedural organization of emotions: A contribution from cognitive science to the psychoanalytic theory of therapeutic action. *J. Amer. Psychoanal. Assn.,* 39:349–382.

Cohen, N. J. & Squire, L. R. (1980), Preserved learning and retention of pattern-analyzing skill in amnesia. Dissociation of knowing how and knowing that. *Science,* 210:207–210.

Craik, K. (1943), *The Nature of Explanation.* Cambridge, UK: Cambridge University Press.

Crockenberg, S. & Litman, C. (1990), Autonomy as competence in two-year-olds: Maternal correlates of child compliance, defiance, and self-assertion. *Devel. Psychol.,* 26:961–971.

Damasio, A. (1994), *Descartes' Error: Emotion, Reason and the Human Brain.* New York: Putnam.

Edelman, G. M. (1987), *Neural Darwinism.* New York: Basic Books.

Fairbairn, W. R. D. (1952), *An Object-Relations Theory of the Personality.* New York: Basic Books.

Fischer, K. (1980), A theory of cognitive development: The control and construction of hierarchies of skills. *Psychol. Bull.*, 87:477–531.

Fischer, K. & Granott, N. (1995), Beyond one-dimensional change: Parallel, concurrent, socially distributed processes in learning and development. *Human Devel.*, 38:302–314.

—— & Pipp, S. (1984), Development of structures of unconscious thought. In: *The Unconscious Reconsidered*, ed. K. Bowers & D. Meichenbaum. New York: Wiley, pp. 88–148.

—— & Watson, M. (1981), Explaining the Oedipus conflict. *Cognitive Development*, 12:79–92.

Fonagy, P. (1991), Thinking about thinking: Some clinical and theoretical considerations in the treatment of the borderline patient. *Internat. J. Psycho-Anal.*, 72:639–656.

Freeman, W. (1990), Searching for signal and noise in the chaos of brain waves. In: *The Ubiquity of Chaos*, ed. S. Krasner. Washington, DC: American Association for the Advancement of Science, pp. 47–55.

Grice, H. P. (1975), Logic and conversation. In: *Syntax and Semantics III: Speech Acts*, ed. P. Lole & J. L. Moran. New York: Academic Press, pp. 41–58.

Gunnar, M., Brodersen, L., Nachmias, M., Buss, K. & Rigatuso, R. (in press), Stress reactivity and attachment security. *Devel. Psychobiol.*

Hertsgaard, L., Gunnar, M., Erickson, M. & Nachmias, M. (1995), Adrenocortical response to the strange situation in infants with disorganized/disoriented attachment relationships. *Child Devel.*, 66:1100–1106.

Hobson, P. (1993), The intersubjective domain: Approaches from developmental psychopathology. *J. Amer. Psychoanal. Assn. Suppl. Research*, 61:167–192.

Hoffman, I. (1992), Some practical implications of a social constructivist view of the psychoanalytic situation. *Psychoanal. Dial.*, 2:287–304.

Izard, C. E. (1978), Emotions as motivation: An evolutionary–developmental perspective. In: *Nebraska Symposium on Motivation*, ed. R. A. Dienstbier. Lincoln, NE: University of Nebraska Press, pp. 163–200.

Jacobs, T. (1991), The interplay of enactments: Their role in the analytic process. In: *The Use of the Self*, ed. T. Jacobs. Madison, CT: International Universities Press, pp. 31–49.

Jacoby, L. L. & Dallas, M. (1981), On the relationship between autobiographical memory and perceptual learning. *J. Exper. Psychol.: Gen.*, 110:300–324.

Kernberg, O. (1976), *Object Relations Theory and Clinical Psychoanalysis*. New York: Aronson.

Kihlstrom, J. (1987), The cognitive unconscious. *Science*, 237:1445–1452.

Kobak, R. & Sceery, A. (1988), Attachment in late adolescence: Working models, affect regulation, and representations of self and others. *Child Devel.*, 59:135–146.

Landry, M. & Lyons-Ruth, K. (1980), Recursive structure in cognitive perspective-taking. *Child Devel.*, 51:386–394.

Lewis, M. (1995), Memory and psychoanalysis: A new look at infantile amnesia and transference. *J. Amer. Acad. Child Adol. Psychiat.*, 34:405–417.

Lichtenberg, J. (1989), *Psychoanalysis and Motivation*. Hillsdale, NJ: The Analytic Press.

Lyons-Ruth, K. (1991), Rapprochement or approchement: Mahler's theory reconsidered from the vantage point of recent research on early attachment relationships. *Psychoanal. Psychol.*, 8:1–23.

———— (1998), Implicit relational knowing: Its role in development and psychoanalytic treatment. *Infant Mental Health J.,* 19:282–289.

———— (in press), "I sense that you sense that I sense . . .": Sander's recognition process and implicit relational knowing in the psychotherapeutic setting. *Infant Mental Health J., Festschrift Issue in Honor of Dr. Louis Sander.*

———— Alpern, L. & Repacholi, B. (1993), Disorganized infant attachment classification and maternal psychosocial problems as predictors of hostile-aggressive behavior in the preschool classroom. *Child Devel.,* 64:572–585.

———— Bronfman, E. & Atwood, G. (1999), A relational diathesis model of hostile-helpless states of mind: Expressions in mother–infant interaction. In: *Attachment Disorganization,* ed. J. Solomon & C. George. New York: Guilford, pp. 33–70.

———— Bronfman, E. & Parsons, E. (1999), Maternal disrupted affective communication, maternal frightened or frightening behavior, and disorganized infant attachment strategies. In: *Atypical Patterns of Infant Attachment: Theory, Research and Current Directions,* ed. J. Vondra & D. Barnett. *Monographs of the Society for Research in Child Development,* 64.

———— & Zeanah, C. (1993), The family context of infant mental health, Part I: Affective development in the primary caregiving relationship. In: *Handbook of Infant Mental Health,* ed. C. Zeanah. New York: Guilford, 1993, pp. 14–26.

———— & Jacobvitz, D. (1999), Attachment disorganization: Unresolved loss, relational violence, and lapses in behavioral and attentional strategies. In: *Handbook of Attachment Theory and Research,* ed. J. Cassidy and P. Shaver. New York: Guilford, pp. 520–554.

Main, M. (1993), Discourse, prediction, and recent studies in attachment: Implications for psychoanalysis. *J. Amer. Psychoanal. Assn., Suppl. on Res. in Psychoanal.,* 61:209–243.

———— & Goldwyn, R. (1994), Adult Attachment Rating and Classification System. Unpublished coding manual, Department of Psychology, University of California at Berkeley, Berkeley, CA.

———— & Hesse, E. (1990), Parents' unresolved traumatic experiences are related to infant disorganized attachment status: Is frightened and/or frightening parental behavior the linking mechanism? In: *Attachment in the Preschool Years: Theory, Research and Intervention,* ed. M. Greenberg, D. Cicchetti, & E. M. Cummings. Chicago: University of Chicago Press, pp. 161–184.

———— Kaplan, N. & Cassidy, J. (1985), Security in infancy, childhood and adulthood: A move to the level of representation. In: *Growing Points of Attachment Theory and Research. Monographs of the Society for Research in Child Development,* ed. I. Bretherton & E. Waters. 50:66–104.

———— Tomasini, L. & Tolan, W. (1979), Differences among mothers of infants judged to differ in security of attachment. *Devel. Psychol.,* 15:472–473.

Malatesta, C. Z., Culber, C., Tesman, J. R. & Shepard, B. (1989), The development of emotion expression during the first two years of life. *Monogr. Soc. Res. Child Devel.,* 54.

Marcel, A. (1983), Conscious and unconscious perception: Experiments on visual masking and word recognition. *Cognitive Psychol.,* 15:197–237.

McLaughlin, J. (1991), Clinical and theoretical aspects of enactment. *J. Amer. Psychoanal. Assn.,* 39:595–614.

Mitchell, S. (1988), *Relational Concepts in Psychoanalysis.* Cambridge, MA: Harvard University Press.

Ogden, T. (1994), The analytic third: Working with intersubjective clinical facts. *Internat. J. Psycho-Anal.*, 75:3–19.

Oster, H., & Eckman, P. (1977), Facial behavior in child development. In: *Minnesota Symnposium on Child Psychology*, Vol. 11, ed. A. Collins. New York: Thomas A. Crowell, pp. 231–376.

Piaget, J. & Inhelder, B. (1973), *Memory and Intelligence*. New York: Basic Books.

Prigogine, I. & Stengers, I. (1984), *Order Out of Chaos: Man's New Dialogue with Nature*. New York: Bantam Books.

Rumelhart, D. E., & McClelland, J. L. & the PDP Research Group. (1986), *Parallel Distributed Processing, Vol. 1*. Cambridge: MIT Press.

Sander, L. (1987), Awareness of inner experience: A systems perspective on self-regulatory process in early development. *Child Abuse and Neglect.*, 11:339–346.

————— (1995), Thinking about developmental process: Wholeness, specificity, and the organization of conscious experiencing. Invited address, annual meeting of the Division of Psychoanalysis, American Psychological Association. Santa Monica, CA.

Sandler, J. & Sandler, A. (1994), The past unconscious and the present unconscious: A contribution to a technical frame of reference. *The Psychoanalytic Study of the Child*, 49:278–292. New Haven, CT: Yale University Press.

Schacter, D. L. & Buckner, R. L. (1998), Priming and the brain. *Neuron,* 20:185–195.

————— & Moscovitch, M. (1984), Infants, amnesia and dissociable memory systems. In: *Infant Memory*, ed. M. Moscovitch. New York: Plenum, pp. 173–216.

Seligman, S. (1995), Applying infant observation research to psychoanalytic clinical work: A contemporary perspective. Plenary presentation to the Congress of the International Psychoanalytic Studies Organization of the International Psychoanalytical Association. San Francisco, July.

Selman, R. F. (1980), *The Growth of Interpersonal Understanding*. New York: Academic Press.

Spangler, G. & Grossmann, K. E. (1993), Biobehavioral organization in securely and insecurely attached infants. *Child Devel.*, 64:1439–1450.

Stern, D. (1998), The process of therapeutic change involving implicit knowledge: Some implications of developmental observations for adult psychotherapy. *Infant Mental Health J.,* 19:300–308.

————— (1985), *The Interpersonal World of the Infant: A View from Psychoanalysis and Developmental Psychology*. New York: Basic Books.

————— (1995), *The Motherhood Constellation*. New York: Basic Books.

————— Sander, L., Nahum, J., Harrison, A., Lyons-Ruth, K., Morgan, A., Bruschweiler-Stern, N. & Tronick, E. Z. (1998), Non-interpretive mechanisms in psychoanalytic therapy: The "something more" than interpretation. *Internat. J. Psycho-Anal.*, 79:903–921.

Stolorow, R. (in press), Dynamic, dyadic, intersubjective systems: An evolving paradigm for psychoanalysis. *Internat. J. Psycho. Anal.*

Thelen, E. & Smith, L. B. (1994), *A Dynamic Systems Approach to the Development of Cognition and Action*. Cambridge: MIT Press/Bradford Books.

Trevarthen C (1980), The foundations of intersubjectivity: Development of interpersonal and cooperative understanding in infants. In: *The Social Foundations of Language and Thought*, ed. D. Olson. New York: Norton, pp. 316–342.

Tronick, E. (1989), Emotions and emotional communication in infants. *Amer. Psychol.*, 44:112–119.

——— (1998), Dyadically expanded states of consciousness and the process of normal and abnormal development. *Infant Mental Health J.*, 19:300–308.

Tulving, E. (1972), Episodic and semantic memory. In: *Organization of Memory*, ed. E. Tulving & W. Donaldson. New York: Academic Press, pp. 382–403.

van IJzendoorn, M. H. (1995), Adult attachment representations, parental responsiveness, and infant attachment: A meta-analysis on the predictive validity of the Adult Attachment Interview. *Psychol. Bull.*, 117:387–403.

Vygotsky, L. S. (1962), *Thought and Language*. Cambridge: MIT Press.

Westen, D. (1990), Towards a revised theory of borderline object relations: Contributions of empirical research. *Internat. J. Psycho-Anal.*, 71:661–694.

Wolff, P. (1996), The irrelevance of infant observations for psychoanalysis. *J. Amer. Psychoanal. Assn.*, 44:369–391.

Wood, D., Bruner, J. & Ross, G. (1976), The role of tutoring in problem-solving. *J. Child Psychol. & Psychiat.*, 17:89–100.

Department of Psychiatry
Cambridge Hospital
1493 Cambridge Street
Cambridge, MA 02139

The Development of Caregiving:
A Comparison of Attachment Theory and
Psychoanalytic Approaches to Mothering

CAROL GEORGE, Ph.D.
JUDITH SOLOMON, Ph.D.

"Do not ride your bicycle around the corner," the mother had told
the daughter when she was seven. "Why not?" protested the girl.
"Because then I cannot see you and you will fall down and cry
and I will not hear you." "How do you know I'll fall?" whined
the girl. "It is in the book, The Twenty Six Malignant Gates, all
of the bad things that can happen to you outside the protection of
this house." . . . It would have been enough to think that even one
of these dangers could befall a child . . . my mother worried
about them all. . . . So by taking them all into account, she had
absolute faith she could prevent every one of them.

Amy Tan, *The Joy Luck Club*

Hush now baby don't you cry.
Mama's gonna make all your nightmares come true,
Mama's gonna put all her fears into you.
Mama's gonna keep you right under her wing,
She won't let you fly but she might let you sing.

Dr. George is a member of the Department of Psychology, Mills College, Oakland, CA.
Dr. Solomon is a member of the Center for the Family in Transition, Corte Madera, CA. We
would like to thank Malcolm West for his comments on earlier drafts of this paper. This work
was supported in part by the Letts-Villard Endowed Chair in the Sciences awarded to the first
author. Address correspondence to Carol George.

Mama will keep you cozy and warm.
Ooooh Baby, of course, mom'll help build the wall.

Roger Waters, "Mother," from *The Wall*

A TTACHMENT THEORY AND PSYCHOANALYSIS ARE FOUNDED on the premise of the ultimate importance of mothering. Both theoretical traditions emphasize that the sensitive, responsive, empathic mother who is behaviorally or intrapsychically attuned to her child fosters development and helps buffer her child from psychopathology. In contrast, the insensitive, narcissistic, or unempathic mother is seen as placing the child at developmental and pathological risk. Despite the shared emphasis on the importance of the mother, these traditions have approached mothering almost exclusively in terms of the psychological experience of the *child*. Little attention has been paid in either tradition to the fact that mothering has its own developmental trajectory and is a separate, autonomous motivational system.

Attachment theory conceives of maternal behavior as motivated and organized by the caregiving behavioral system. Bowlby (1969) described the caregiving system only briefly in his writing, however, and there has been little effort to expand on this aspect of attachment theory. Following trends long established in developmental psychology and guided by the empirical methodology of psychological science, the mother in attachment research typically is treated as a variable—a set of discrete behavioral or qualitative dimensions. Although recently there has been greater interest in the "parental side of attachment" (e.g., Aber et al., 1989; Bretherton, et al., 1989; Zeanah et al., 1995; Slade et al., 1997), this research has not been concerned with understanding the organization of attachment and caregiving as distinct, complementary motivational systems.

A unique feature of our work is our examination of caregiving as an organized motivational system in its own right, linked developmentally and behaviorally to attachment (George and Solomon, 1989, 1996, 1999; Solomon and George, 1996, 1999a). In this paper we summarize our thinking regarding caregiving, highlighting points of convergence and divergence between the attachment and psychoanalytic traditions. (For a comprehensive review of the interface between attachment and psychoanalysis, see Ammaniti and Stern, 1992; Slade and Aber, 1992; Diamond and Blatt, 1994.) We begin our discussion with a historical overview of attachment theory and psychoanalytic approaches to mothering. We then describe mothering more fully through the unique lens derived from attachment theory—the caregiving behavioral system.

Attachment Theory and Psychoanalysis: Historical Overview of Mothering

A central feature of caregiving that emerges in both traditions is the mother's ability to evaluate the child's developmental status and attune to the child's rhythms and needs. The emphasis of attachment theory and research on mothering is consistent with contemporary psychoanalytic approaches; both emphasize the interrelatedness between mother and child, the importance of environmental factors as major influences on development, and child pathology and developmental risk as related to maternal failure in the early years (Eagle, 1995). The mother is viewed as crucial in supporting age-appropriate development in the child (e.g., Sroufe, 1979; Solomon, George, and Ivins, 1987; Crittenden, 1995), including emotional attunement and empathy (Winnicott, 1958; Emde, Gaensbauer, and Harmon, 1976; Sroufe, 1979; Stern, 1985; Tronick, 1989). Further, the mother–infant bond is viewed in both traditions as fundamental to the quality of the child's later relationships (Bowlby, 1969, 1988; Mahler, Pine, and Bergman, 1975; Main, Kaplan, and Cassidy, 1985; Ainsworth, 1989; Thompson, 1999) and the stability and coherence of the self (Winnicott, 1958; Bowlby, 1969, 1980; Mahler et al., 1975; Emde, Gaensbauer, and Harman, 1976; Cassidy and Kobak, 1988; Main, 1990; Cassidy, 1994; Carlson, 1998).

Historically, however, there have also been important differences in how the two traditions have viewed mothering. Detailed descriptions of maternal behavior have been a primary component of attachment theory and research from its inception. Bowlby's original conceptualization of attachment emphasized the behavior of the attachment figure as reciprocal and complementary to the infant's attachment behavior (Bowlby, 1969; 1980). During Bowlby's era, developmental research depicted the early capabilities and achievements of human infants. Bowlby (1969), thus viewed the infant as primed toward interaction and seeking contact with attachment figures and the mother as an active dyadic partner beginning at birth. Attachment theory's empirical approach to mothering is tied to Ainsworth's definition of attachment security. Ainsworth described mothering in terms of four broad interactive components. Chief among these was maternal sensitivity, defined as prompt and appropriate response to infant signals. Maternal acceptance, psychological availability, and cooperativeness were highly intercorrelated with sensitivity (Ainsworth et al., 1978). Three decades of research have demonstrated that mothers who provide sensitive and responsive care foster secure attachment and age-appropriate development; mothers who are insensitive, intrusive, or rejecting foster insecure attachment and compromise development (see Thompson, 1999; cf., Solomon and George, 1999).

In contrast to attachment theory, there was little original interest in describing mothering in psychoanalysis. As compared with the robust attachment infant, the drive theory infant was depicted as in a state of primary narcissism, that is, the infant experiences him- or herself as self-sufficient and therefore has no need for a mothering figure. Indeed, the mother is not truly an object (i.e., a person) for the infant but simply a vehicle for drive gratification. The object becomes a mother figure to the young infant through feeding interactions, or what Bowlby described as the "cupboard theory of mothering" (Bowlby, 1969). Descriptions of the mother herself, then, were relatively absent in traditional drive theory. Cohen, Cohler, and Weissman (1984) explained, "Parenthood for Freud, after he renounced the seduction hypothesis for the development of neurosis, was not a major area of interest" (p. 263).

Object relations theories shifted the focus of infant development from feeding to social interaction, as captured by Fairbairn's (1952) well-known proposition that the infant is not pleasure-seeking but rather object-seeking. The fundamental goal of the mother was to support individuation (Mahler et al., 1975), independence (Winnicott, 1958), or the development of an integrated self (Fairbairn, 1952). Thus, in the object relations view the mother was elevated to an esteemed position. As with attachment theory, object relations theories articulated mothering in terms of what was optimal from the infant's point of view. Unlike the observation-based descriptions of the attachment theory mother, object relations descriptions were derived from clinical experience and emphasized the subjective experience of mothering.

The first systematic psychoanalytic interest in mothering appeared in Benedek's (1959; Anthony and Benedek, 1970) seminal work on parenthood. Benedek emphasized the development of the mother herself, in particular, important transformations of the self during pregnancy. We see the theme of parental transformation emerge again later in Kohut's self-theory (Kohut and Wolff, 1978). In contrast to Benedict, Kohut added to the concept of mothering the importance of making the child the center of her perception and modulating against the intrusion of her own inner conflicts (Kohut and Wolf, 1978; Elson, 1984).

Two new strands of interest in mothering have begun to emerge in psychoanalysis. One strand follows Benedek's and Kohut's approach to parenthood as a phase or developmental process (Cohen et al., 1984). Some theorists in this strand have adopted a life-span view, emphasizing the contribution of parental experiences with children at different ages to the development of the self (e.g., Elson, 1984; Schwartz, 1984). Other theorists have focused on the transition to parenthood as a "life crisis" precipitated by pregnancy (e.g., Bibring et al., 1961; Deutscher, 1971; Liefer, 1980; Ammaniti, 1994; Lee, 1995) and accompanied by processes of parental separation and individuation (Diamond, Heinicke, and Mintz, 1996). Another strand of neo-psychoanalysts have begun to flesh out in more detail than their early object relations counterparts the intrapsychic aspects of mothering (e.g., Emde et al., 1976; Stern, 1985; Stern-Bruschweiler and Stern, 1989; Emde, 1994; Sandler, 1994). These new strands not only emphasize the importance of mothering, but also begin to add normative, research-based descriptions of mothering to the psychoanalytic tradition.

As we examine the approaches toward mothering of these two disciplines today, we see more similarities than differences. Although qualitatively distinct, both view the mother as important and describe her in terms of how well or how badly she meets the child's needs. Attachment theory continues to emphasize empirical descriptions of mothering over intrapsychic ones, although the field's move to the level of representation has brought the two traditions closer in this regard as well. Psychoanalytic theory continues to emphasize the intrapsychic aspects of mothering, although, as mentioned above, psychoanalytic studies are beginning to adopt an empirical approach to research. Despite these similarities, attachment theory offers a unique contribution to our understanding of mothering. It calls our attention to the instinctual, goal-directed nature of caregiving, that is, to the biological substrate and evolution of maternal behavior. We will argue that the caregiving behavioral system fundamentally organizes and regulates caregiving behavior, a function that is basic to survival and reproductive fitness and one of most powerful of human experiences, with profound implications for both caregiver and child. The remainder of our discussion focuses on this contribution—an ethological behavioral systems approach to caregiving.

An Ethological Approach to Caregiving: The Caregiving Behavioral System

Bowlby (1969) adopted an ethological approach to attachment and caregiving based on two strong convictions. One conviction was that certain essential behaviors, such as those related to seeking and providing care, were expressions of independent, instinctual motivational systems related to adaptation, survival, and reproductive fitness. This view permits the examination of discrete patterns of behavior in relation to their adaptive function; it contrasts with the traditional libido theory position that behavior represents varying expressions of a single drive (Bowlby, 1984). The other conviction was that individual differences in behavior were the product of individual differences in real experience. Thus, by adopting the ethological perspective, Bowlby soundly rejected psychoanalytic models (drive and object relations theories) that conceived of behavior as primarily the product of intrapsychic conflict and fantasy. While Bowlby (1969) made ethological principles the foundation of his theory, the field, as it has evolved, has come increasingly to emphasize attachment as a model of child and, more recently, adult mental health. The ethological components of Bowlby's original model are often left behind in this endeavor. With regard to mothering, the ethological or behavioral systems perspective seems never to have been clearly adopted.

Behavioral systems are believed to organize a large repertoire of behavior in humans and other species, including attachment, parenting, sexual, affiliative, exploratory, feeding, and wariness (Hinde, 1982). Bowlby stressed that the mother–child relationship was organized in terms of co-adapted behavioral systems. "Behaviour complementary to attachment behaviour and serving a complementary function, that of protecting the attached individual, is caregiving. This is commonly shown by a parent, or other adult, towards a child or adolescent" (Bowlby, 1980, p. 40). There are several tenets of behavioral systems that we wish to emphasize here as especially important to our discussion of the caregiving system.

(1) *Behavior that is tied to a specific behavioral system is organized and goal-corrected.* That is, goals extend over long periods of time, and the behaviors needed to achieve those goals are adjusted flexibly, in a nonrandom fashion, to a wide range of environments and to the development of the individual (Bowlby, 1969). Behavioral adjustments are regulated by a biological feedback system that monitors internal (central nervous system activity, hormones) and environmental cues leading to the system's activation or termination.

(2) *The individual's survival and reproductive fitness depends on having an appropriately balanced repertoire of instinctive behavioral systems that together influence behavior.* Not all systems are activated simultaneously; the organism monitors and responds to the activation and termination of an integrated set of systems. In some instances the simultaneous activation of two or more systems may lead to conflicting or incompatible behavior. Note that this premise fits well with psychoanalytic postulates regarding conflict in relation to the complex interplay of motivational forces. The major difference in the two perspectives lies in the proposed source, functions, and goals of the motivation.

(3) *Some systems begin as nonfunctional and become functional as they are integrated with other systems.* This is especially evident with regard to adult behavioral systems. Isolated movements or behavior related to adult systems appear in incomplete forms during childhood yet do not become integrated into organized behavioral sequences until the

individual experiences developmentally appropriate catalysts for their maturation.

(4) *At least in primates, behavioral systems are regulated in the mind by cognitive models that evaluate and organize the organism's experience and affective appraisal.* These models are updated and reworked to achieve internal consistency and are available for use in novel situations or as the basis of constructing future plans.

(5) *The behavioral sequences governed by behavioral systems are influenced by the idiosyncrasies of environmental or contextual variables.* "Because of a human's capacity to learn and to develop complex behavioral systems, it is usual for his instinctive behavior to become incorporated into flexible behavioral sequences that vary from individual to individual" (Bowlby, 1969, p. 160), thus, explaining the lability of behavioral systems and the wide range of individual differ ences in human behavior that achieve the same proximate goal. Hinde (1982), and later Main (1990), emphasized that in some environments the organism develops conditional strategies that are manipulations of the primary expression of a behavioral system.

We begin our discussion with the first two points. The evolutionary function of the attachment and caregiving systems is protection of the young; the proximate goal of both attachment and caregiving behavior is to seek and maintain proximity. Although the caregiving and attachment systems are reciprocal, goal-corrected behavior guided by these two systems is not organized in identical ways. Thus, defining the caregiving system requires a shift in thinking away from the child to the parent, a point that is echoed in some psychoanalytic perspectives on mothering (e.g., Kohut and Wolf, 1978; Elson, 1984; Sadow, 1984). The important difference between attachment and caregiving is that the child's attachment system is organized to *seek* protection from the attachment figure; in contrast, the caregiving system is organized to *provide* protection for the child. The shift may seem obvious when delineated in this fashion; however, this emphasis on the parent as the one who provides protection has not been integrated fully into attachment theory or other models of parental behavior (e.g., discussions of caregiving in terms of "parental attachment"; Bretherton et al., 1989). Certainly parental behavior characterized by sensitivity, responsiveness, perspective-taking, or empathy contribute meaningfully to the child's attachment security, but there are advantages to considering these and other classes of parental behavior and thought in terms of a caregiving system organized fundamentally around the goal of providing protection. Thus, from the perspective of the caregiver, the question can be posed, "How does sensitivity to the infant's signals permit the mother to fulfill her goal of protection?" We suggest that the answer to this may be that the baby's signals are one source of reasonably reliable cues as to when her care or protection is needed and what sort of care is called for, allowing her efficiently to minister to her infant or to turn her attention elsewhere as appropriate.

Drawing upon the second tenet of behavioral systems, defining the caregiving system also requires an expanded view of the parent, one that requires the consideration of how caregiving is integrated within the mother's full repertoire of adult behavioral systems, particularly those that compete with caregiving. Bowlby (1969) describes the mother–child relationship as comprised of the general classes of behavior that include the child's attachment behavior and behavior antithetic to attachment, and the mother's caregiving behavior and behavior antithetic to caregiving. With regard to antithetical child behavioral systems, researchers have predominantly described attachment in relation to the exploratory system. Classification of attachment security based on behavior in the Strange Situation (Ainsworth et al., 1978) and in the home is largely based on an evaluation of the balance of the attachment and exploratory systems (Waters and Deane, 1985). With regard to mothering, although Bowlby implies that mothers have life demands that compete with providing protection and care for the child, he more frequently writes as if the mother's desire to provide protection and the child's desire to be protected overlap completely. This view is consistent with developmental psychology and psychoanalytic views of mothering, views that are guided implicitly, and often explicitly, by the principle that "good" mothers are always sensitive to their infants and "bad" or inadequate mothers are not. In reality, parent and child have some overlapping interests, and as Trivers (1974) pointed out, there are also evolutionary-based conflicts between them.

Thus, at both the proximate and ultimate levels, the level and quality of caregiving can be expected to reflect a kind of balance among competing activities and imperatives. At the proximate level, the caregiving system, although a very important and powerful adult motivational system, is not the only system that determines a mother's behavior (Stevenson-Hinde, 1994). Just as the infant must seek a dynamic balance between its behavioral systems, the mother must strike a balance between her desire to protect and nurture the child and other needs and goals. Consider for a moment caregiving in relation to other relationship-based behavioral systems. Competing with caregiving is the mother's sexual relationship with her partner, affiliative relationships and friendships, and her own protection needs (i.e., attachment). The balance struck by the mother among these and other competing motivational systems is likely to reflect a variety of contextual influences, including the support given to her in her role as mother, demands by others, cultural mores, the requirements of a particular child, her own childhood and adult attachment experiences, and her experiences as a caregiver of each of her children. These factors taken together will influence her perception of danger and safety and her ability and willingness to provide protection for a particular child.

At the ultimate, or evolutionary, level, the fundamental goal of all mothers is reproductive fitness. In order to maximize her fitness the mother must raise a child to become an independent, fully functioning adult. The sooner the child begins to demonstrate independence, however, the sooner the mother can invest in other offspring or in other goals related to her survival and fitness. The optimal caregiving strategy, therefore, requires the mother to be flexible in relation to both her other goals and the developmental status of the child (Solomon and George, 1996). Flexible caregiving appears to be characteristic of mothers in most societies; under difficult environmental conditions, this pattern seems to grant distinct selective advantages to the child (Kermoian and Liederman, 1986; True, 1994). Under other conditions, however, alternative caregiving strategies may be more advantageous to the mother. Logically, mothers can choose from a range of strategies, including protection of the child from a distance (promoting greater independence at earlier ages) or protection by keeping the child close (encouraging greater dependence on her).

Once we begin to look at caregiving from the mother's perspective, we see the issue of "good enough" or "bad" mothering in a new light. Maternal care should support the mother's lifetime reproductive fitness, and in *evolutionary* terms, strategies that broadly support this goal can be defined as "good enough." "Good enough" caregiving, thus, may be defined as caregiving that is fundamentally organized around protection of the child, with the longer-term outcome of permitting the child to reproduce successfully (i.e., contribute to the mother's fitness). Thus, the mother who abdicates her role as the child's protector either consistently or intermittently may be said to fail to meet the standards of "good enough" mothering. Practically speaking, mothering would be considered good enough if it supports development in such a way that the child is not placed at developmental or pathological risk. This definition, based on functional considerations, is impartial with respect to developmental cost and psychological stress to the child as long as these do not overwhelm the child's capacity for adaptation, that is, is not associated with serious maladaptation. (For another perspective on "good enough" maternal strategies derived from evolutionary considerations, see Belsky [1999]).

The notion of good enough mothering is itself derived from Winnicott's object relations approach (1958). Building upon this work, Schwartz (1984) noted that the average expectable parent is inherently imperfect and must only provide what is required at each stage of development. The concept of good enough mothering is more foreign to attachment theory, which has emphasized maternal behavior in relation to the child's optimal development (in typical, low-stress childrearing conditions, and only in a fairly narrow range of human cultures). Mothering that results in anything less than optimal development in the child is not considered good enough from the attachment perspective. Historically, mothering that is not good enough has included mothering associated with traditionally insecure attachment (avoidant and ambivalent attachment). Early research showed that traditional forms of insecurity, particularly avoidance, appeared to compromise some aspects of development (e.g., self-esteem, ego-integrity, cooperation—see reviews by Sroufe, 1988;

Cicchetti and Carlson, 1989; Greenberg, Cicchetti, and Cummings, 1990; Thompson, 1999). Recent studies that include the disorganized attachment category suggest, however, that it is this group and not the traditional insecure groups that is associated with appreciable behavioral maladjustment (Moss et al., in press; Lyons-Ruth, 1996; Lyons-Ruth and Block, 1996; Moss et al., 1996, in press; Carlson 1998; Solomon and George, 1996b; Moss et al., 1998). These findings are consistent with our conclusions based on extensive interview and observation of mothers whose children are classified into one of the four attachment groups (secure, avoidant, ambivalent, or disorganized/controlling) (George and Solomon, 1996; Solomon, George, and Silverman, in press). Despite important qualitative differences, the caregiving of mothers of children classified as secure or insecure-avoidant or ambivalent are all organized around the fundamental goal of protection. Only the mothers of children in the disorganized group can be said to show serious lapses in their protective orientation toward their children. We will return to this topic in a later section when we examine the caregiving representations and child risk.

Ontogeny of Caregiving

In the attachment, as well as the psychoanalytic traditions the young child is believed to develop both a sense of receiving care and of providing care in the context of his or her early relationships, which is carried forward into new relationships (Bretherton, 1985; Sroufe and Fleeson, 1986). Indeed, in attachment theory (Bowlby, 1973, 1980; Sroufe and Fleeson, 1986), social learning theory, and psychoanalysis (Benedek, 1959; see also Fonagy, 1994) psychologists have conceived of mothering almost exclusively in terms of intergenerational transmission of a woman's behavioral model or intrapsychic representation of her own mother. This view has been endorsed by a growing number of attachment theorists and supported by research comparing the mother's adult attachment with that of the child (Bretherton, 1985; Main et al., 1985; Grossmann et al., 1988; Haft and Slade, 1989; Ainsworth and Eichberg, 1991; Fonagy, Steele, and Steele, 1991; Ward et al., 1991; Bus and van IJzendoorn, 1992; Benoit and Parker, 1994; Fonagy et al., 1995; Main, 1995; Slade et al., 1995; van IJzendoorn, 1995). There can be little doubt for primates in general, and for humans in particular, that early experience of being mothered is a necessary condition for the later expression of adequately organized caregiving (Fraiberg, 1980; Fleming, Corter, and Steiner, 1995; Pryce, 1995; Lyons-Ruth and Block, 1996). At the same time, there is a growing body of literature—clinical, comparative, and developmental—to suggest that early experience is neither a sufficient nor a final determinant of the quality of later caregiving.

Within the attachment literature proper, recent findings suggest both less continuity over time in an individual's attachment security (see e.g., Belsky et al., 1996) and a more complex picture with respect to intergenerational continuity than anticipated by theory. The mechanism by which intergenerational continuity of the attachment-caregiving system might be achieved is also obscure at this time. Bowlby (1969), and later Main (1990), proposed that maternal sensitivity was the mechanism of transmission from mother to child. Meta-analyses of a range of studies on maternal sensitivity have shown, however, that sensitivity only accounts for a small percentage of the variance between maternal caregiving and the child's attachment (van IJzendoorn, 1995; de Wolf and van IJzendoorn, 1997).

As we have discussed fully elsewhere (Solomon and George, 1996; George and Solomon, 1999), the strongest tests to date of intergenerational transmission of caregiving are found in several studies that have examined whether the mother's state of mind regarding attachment (as assessed using the AAI; George, Kaplan, and Main, 1984/1985/1996) predict the quality of her infant's later attachment to her (Fonagy et al., 1991; Benoit and Parker, 1994; Slade et al., 1995; Zeanah et al., 1995; George and Solomon, 1996). These studies have reported significant congruence between the mother's attachment security and the child's, but mainly for mothers classified prenatally as secure (Slade et al., 1995). Discrepancies between maternal and infant attachment indicated that mothers classified prenatally as insecure were more likely to have secure infants than the reverse. One interpretation of these findings is that the experiences of pregnancy and parturition, along with experiences with the actual infant, tend to favor the consolidation of a flexible, sensitive caregiving style (Fonagy et al., 1991; Benoit and Parker, 1994; Slade et al., 1995; Zeanah et al., 1995; George and Solomon, 1996).

Discontinuities in attachment within and across generations are less surprising when this issue is approached from the perspective of the ontogeny and determinants of caregiving itself. While the caregiving system may have its roots developmentally in the construction of working models of self and other in the context of attachment relationships during childhood, under normal conditions, there is reason to believe that the caregiving system is regulated on the cognitive level by a distinct model of relationships with its own developmental trajectory and mental organization. Drawing on the third tenet of behavioral systems described earlier in this paper, the caregiving system would be expected to begin to develop during childhood with the emergence of isolated, immature, nonfunctional forms of caregiving behavior. There is little research on caregiving behavior during the childhood years. Under normal childrearing conditions (i.e., conditions that do not demand a child to take real responsibility for providing care and protection) we propose that the caregiving system remains in an immature form until adolescence (George and Solomon, 1996, 1999; Solomon and George, 1996). It is likely that elements of the caregiving repertoire are first exhibited as early as toddlerhood (and in juveniles of other species) in the form of "play-mothering" as expressed toward babies, including dolls, and animals (Pryce, 1995). During puberty, a time when children make the transition to become biologically capable of bearing children, as with other species, it is likely that the hormonal and neurological changes of this period combine with external stimuli and previous experience to form a sensitive period that initiates transformations in the caregiving system toward maturity.

The caregiving system probably undergoes its greatest development during the transition to parenthood (pregnancy, birth, and the months following birth). Pregnancy could be defined as a life crisis (Lee, 1995) or a bio-social-behavioral shift (Cole and Cole, 1996). At the biological level, pregnancy is accompanied by significant hormonal and neurological changes (Fleming et al., 1995; Pryce, 1995). This is not to suggest that human mothers are dominated by hormones, nor does it undermine the power of human experience and learning, but the influence of these hormones on producing emotional calming and closeness with the infant cannot be discounted. At the cognitive level, we suggest that achievement of formal operational thought and formation of identity contribute to the shift. At the social-emotional level, this period is accompanied by sexual relations, the beginning of responsibility for a new generation, and is often also accompanied by intense emotion and emotional swings that have the potential for both psychological disorganization and a new reorganization of the self (Benedek, 1959; Bibring et al., 1961; Deutscher, 1971; Liefer, 1980; Cowan, 1991; Ammaniti, 1994; Lee, 1995). The shift to caregiving may also be facilitated by the mother's relationships during childbirth itself, including those with the father, medical personnel, and childbirth coaches (Klaus, Kennell, and Klaus, 1995; Manning-Orenstein, 1998).

Of profound importance, in our view, is the power of the baby to elicit caregiving behavior and organize caregiving in the mother. The infant's manifest vulnerability and specific cues are in themselves potent elicitors of protective feelings. Infant characteristics sometimes also present a challenge to caregiving or may even serve as agents of caregiving disorganization (Pianta et al., 1996).

Finally, the social and economic contexts in which the mother finds herself may exert a positive influence on caregiving or may strongly interfere. Marital and social support has been found to enhance mothers' caregiving (Cowan et al., 1991; Belsky, Rosenberger, and Crnic, 1995) while factors such as conflict-laden divorce (Solomon and George, 1999), miscarriage (Slade et al., 1995), and foster care (Stovall and Dozier, 1997) may undermine or disorganize it.

This very brief overview of the ontogeny of caregiving suggests that, in at least some cases, the direction of influence may not be from the past to the present but, rather, the reverse. That is, the mother's caregiving experience may influence, redirect, or confirm how she now views her own childhood attachment experience. In other words, transformations in the caregiving system that result from developmental changes during adolescence, pregnancy, and experiences of being a parent in many cases may serve as catalysts for change. These experiences may facilitate in the mother a reworking of her own behavioral and mental schemes in order to accommodate and integrate new experiences with her infant and herself as a caregiver and protector.

Behavioral Systems and
Organized Representational Models

According to Bowlby, behaviors expressed by behavioral systems are organized by mental or cognitive models. For his conceptualization of mental models, Bowlby (1980) drew upon cognitive theory. The result was a unique attachment theory view of the fundamental psychoanalytic concepts of mental representation, the unconscious, and defense, whereby mental concepts and processes about relationships were explained using the same processes and brain structures that were thought to be involved in processing other kinds of information. Internal working models (Bowlby, 1969, 1973, 1980), representations of interactions that have been generalized (RIGs) (Stern, 1985), and libidinal object constancy (Mahler et al., 1975) all refer to core mental representations. Despite differences in how they are defined, all are seen as exerting their influence out of consciousness, reflecting the importance in both traditions of experience and affect that is processed and/or stored out of awareness.

Attachment theory and psychoanalysis both adhere to the concept of the unconscious and the notion that the majority of the functions of the mind occur out of conscious awareness and the material that "resides" there is incompatible to some degree with the conscious self. They differ, however, in their thinking regarding the nature of this material and the degree to which the unconscious is viewed as determining thought and behavior. In psychoanalysis, the unconscious is a chasm that contains conflict, fear, pain, and guilt that is associated, in particular, with the threatening aspects of the urges, ideas, behavior, or feelings related to sexual and aggressive instincts. This material is forced out of consciousness because it threatens rationality and ego integrity and is thought both directly or indirectly to dominate the individual. Bowlby was only concerned with describing the attachment-related elements of the unconscious. Consistent with psychoanalysis, he viewed the unconscious, nonetheless, as filtering and often limiting partially or fully the negativity associated with memories and experiences. The "dynamic" or overpowering aspects that are implicit to the psychoanalytic unconscious have been removed from the attachment theory concept. Bowlby's (1980) view of the unconscious follows more closely the concept of the nonconscious as defined by cognitive theory. He described the unconscious in terms of more neutral interacting information processing components that work together efficiently and quickly to scan and filter experience, memories, and emotions (a process that has become known in cognitive theory since the time of Bowlby's writing as "parallel distributed processing" [see Kihlstrom, 1990; Westen, 1990]).

The key to the processes of the mind in both the attachment and psychoanalytic traditions is defense. Defensive processes, termed defensive exclusion in attachment theory, shape the form and expression of mental representation and, therefore, behavior in and appraisals of relationships. Defense is invoked to explain processes of the mind that cannot be observed directly but that are inferred from behavior, thought, and affect (Wallerstein, 1983; Kernberg, 1994). Both traditions view defense as linked to satisfying instinctual needs—protecting the individual from breakdown and maladaptation by limiting what is allowed to enter consciousness. In attachment theory, instinctual needs are tied to the activation and deactivation of behavioral systems that serve the basic adaptive function of survival; in psychoanalysis instinctual needs are also linked to survival but in the form of motivational drives (e.g., libido or aggression) that may potentially overwhelm the ego. Certain specific forms of defense are thought to be repeated in similar situations or with certain kinds of relationships (Main, 1990; Kernberg, 1994). Although defensive exclusion has not been studied from a developmental perspective in attachment theory, both traditions propose that the prototypes of defense are established in early childhood in the context of experiences in relationships (Bowlby, 1980; Kernberg, 1994), a view that is mirrored in recent discussions regarding the impact of early relationship trauma on nervous system organization (Perry et al., 1995).

A major difference between psychoanalysis and attachment theory falls in the description of the defensive processes themselves. Contemporary psychoanalytic models utilize a complex constellation of defenses to explain a broad range of intrapsychic phenomenon, including fantasy, dream, wish, and impulse (see, e.g., Horowitz, 1988; Kernberg, 1994). Bowlby (1980), on the other hand, conceived of defensive exclusion in terms of two qualitatively distinct forms of information processing—deactivation and cognitive disconnection.

Deactivation, likened to repression, was defined as the product of systematic scanning, sorting, and excluding information from conscious awareness; deactivation was thought to result in emotional detachment (i.e., isolation of affect). Cognitive disconnection, likened to splitting, was defined as the process of separating affect from the situation or person eliciting it; cognitive deactivation was thought to result in two or more alternative views of the individual or the situation, each view kept separate from the other.

Bowlby proposed that under certain circumstances these two potentially partial forms of exclusion might lead to the development of segregated systems, a pathological form of representation that was organized but kept separate from other representational models and, as much as possible, from conscious awareness. Suggesting that these representational structures developed under conditions of attachment trauma (e.g, unresolved loss of the attachment figure during childhood) he used the concept of segregated systems to explain some forms of relationship-based psychopathology in children and adults. Models that are segregated are necessarily closed to new experience and information and thereby interfere with mental and behavioral health. As defensive exclusion becomes persistent and more complete (i.e., memories and affect walled off from consciousness), the individual is at risk for the sudden emergence or dysregulation of uncontrolled attachment-related material. In this way segregated systems place the individual at risk for psychopathology. Recently, attachment theorists have begun to conceive of certain forms of adult psychopathology such as dissociative disorder in terms of segregated systems (Main and Hesse, 1992; George and West, in press; Liotti, 1999). We will argue later that segregated systems are associated with caregiving risk.

Individual Differences in Maternal Care

Behavioral systems are influenced by the idiosyncrasies of environmental or contextual variables that result in a range of individual differences in caregiving. In our research we have been especially interested in examining individual differences in mother's mental representations of caregiving. We have conceived of these in terms of Bowlby's typology of defensive exclusion and found parallels between mental representations of caregiving and child attachment

(George and Solomon, 1989, 1996; Solomon et al., 1995). Specifically, analysis of interviews during which mothers described their parenting experiences have revealed mental representations that appear to be organized by variations in maternal strategies toward child protection and care and which are associated with characteristic forms of information processing and defense.

The mental representations of mothers of secure children appeared to reflect a strategy of providing direct and flexible care, as revealed in the mothers' descriptions of their behavior and in their frank, forthright (i.e., undefended) discussion of mothering. We found these mothers to be positive and realistic about potential threats to child security; they considered their mothering in relation to the situation, the child's personality and development, their childrearing goals, and their own needs as parents and individuals.

The mental representations of mothers of avoidant and ambivalent children mirrored alternative caregiving strategies, organized around child protection but reflecting a different perception of risks to the child and a different balance in the weight given to mother's and child's needs. Mothers of avoidant children described behavioral strategies of protecting the child from a distance, guided by mild rejection. They evaluated the self and child as somewhat unwilling and unworthy of receiving care and emphasized the negative aspects of their interactions with the child. In terms of defensive processes, the mental representations of mothers of avoidant children were characterized by a partial form of deactivation. These mothers dismissed or devalued their child's attachment needs, thus partially deactivating their caregiving system. Nevertheless, these mothers did not abandon their role in providing care and protection although they tended to focus on physical threats to the child rather than psychological ones. In contrast, mothers of ambivalent children appeared to be uncertain about mothering. They described strategies to keep the child close, appeared insensitive to child cues, and promoted dependency. In terms of defensive processes, the mental representations of uncertain mothers were characterized by a partial form of cognitive disconnection, as revealed by their inability to integrate positive and negative, good and bad, desirable and undesirable. Uncertain and confused, they tended to overemphasize the child's fragility and need for protection from them.

Ontogeny of Developmental Risk:
Abdication of the Caregiving System

In our research, mothers of disorganized or controlling children were characterized by descriptions of the self as helpless to provide care to a child perceived by the mother as beyond control or as mature and self-sufficient (George and Solomon, 1996). These mothers evaluated themselves as lacking effective and appropriate resources to handle caregiving situations and described clear instances in which they abdicated the maternal or protective role toward the child. Helplessness and abdicated care emerged in several forms at the representational level. Most frequently, mothers described themselves or situations with the child where they were psychologically and behaviorally out of control or struggling to remain in control of the circumstances and/or the child. Similarly, they evaluated their child as being out of control (e.g., wild, maniac) or precociously in control of the parent or caregiving situations (e.g., caregiving and role-reversed). Some children were glorified (the child was a gift from God) or described as psychologically merged with the mother ("I am one with this child," "we are connected by an umbilical cord"); some mothers described situations in which maternal care was deemed unnecessary because of special qualities of the child or the relationship. In terms of defense, organized forms of defensive exclusion (i.e., deactivation, cognitive disconnection) were lacking in these interviews. Rather, helplessness was often associated with strong feelings and affective dysregulation. In short, caregiving was disabled in these mothers. They appeared to abdicate their caregiving system, leaving the child unprotected, that is, psychologically or behaviorally abandoned, threatened by the mother or others, or appealed to for reassurance and protection.

We have proposed that the mental representation of caregiving that is characteristic of these mothers can best be conceived in terms of segregated systems and, therefore, subject to being disabled or dysregulated as a result of the experience of helplessness. We suggest that the appraisal of the self as helpless activates the mother's own attachment needs so powerfully that, overwhelmed and perhaps in conflict as to whether to "save" herself or her child, she abdicates caregiving. In these circumstances, the mother's caregiving becomes derailed, so to speak; instead of providing care for the child, she may reach out to the child to fulfill her own attachment needs or unleash deep-seated attachment-related anger or fear (Solomon and George, 1994; West and George, in press). This perception of the self as helpless can arise from a number of potentially interrelated circumstances, including the mother's distorted identification of the infant or child with a previous source of physical danger or psychological trauma (Fraiberg, 1980; Lieberman, 1996); circumstances that the mother believes render her unable to care for or protect him, such as disability (Pianta et al., 1996); divorce (Solomon et al., 1995); unresolved crises or traumatic experiences; or certain kinds of psychopathology (Main and Morgan, 1996).

Conclusions

Our emphasis in this paper was to describe a framework of mothering following the ethological tenets of behavioral systems that are the foundation of attachment theory. It is our hope that this model of the caregiving system contributes to a broader and richer understanding of mothering. This model encompasses the complexity of this fundamental developmental achievement in the adult, which is, at the same time, so important to the developmental achievements of the infant and growing child. We have tried to integrate the major levels of causality—functional, evolutionary, developmental, and immediate— in developing this framework. While we certainly cannot claim to have explicated any one of them fully, our intention has been to outline an approach and to inspire others in the field to consider along with us the many unanswered questions that emerge from it.

In closing, we return here to three defining issues in this area. The first is the nature of the relation between attachment and caregiving. We have suggested that caregiving is regulated by a distinct behavioral system that originates developmentally in the child's experience of primary attachment relationships and, therefore, continues to be linked at the representational level with those experiences. We do not imply that the caregiving system is independent of attachment. Indeed, the experience of being a mother has the potential to evoke continuously memories of the past. By emphasizing the caregiving system, we bring up a point that is obscured in our view in current attachment theory. This point is that, under typical conditions (and these conditions may include stress and hardship), it is expected that the mother will give priority to caregiving, especially when her child is vulnerable or threatened. Further, the mother is expected to give priority to caregiving even when the threat extends to herself, for example, under conditions of domestic violence or environmental catastrophe.

The second issue is the relation between caregiving and the mother's other behavioral systems. Over the past two decades, models of human development have emphasized the transactional and dialectic aspects of developmental processes (see, e.g., Sameroff and Chandler, 1975; Scarr and McCartney, 1983; Blatt and Blass, 1994). Especially important to our thinking about caregiving is the conceptualization of how behavioral systems are integrated and dialectically intertwined during the course of development. We propose that healthy psychological development in the parent may entail not only the transformation from the position of receiving care to that of providing care, but also full integration of the adult repertoire of behavioral systems. This mature integration would serve as the behavioral system foundation of a parent's ability to balance competing needs and ultimately provide good enough care for a child.

The third issue is the notion of "good enough" care. Our operational definition of good enough mothering differs somewhat from that of Winnicott and offers a new approach for consideration when using the attachment framework to interpret maternal behavior. Our point is that, when the mother's perspective and imperatives (developmental and contextual) are considered, good enough can be evaluated along ultimate or proximate dimensions. The ultimate dimension (maternal fitness) is difficult to evaluate in human mothers given current social conditions where birth control, religion, and other social factors have complicated the process of having and caring for babies. The proximate level (maternal and child development), however, is within our grasp as psychologists. There has been little interest in mothers' development with regard to caregiving and their children's attachment, and this is an area that deserves more empirical attention. We are able, however, to evaluate the child's development using the emerging developmental data regarding insecurely attached children (avoidant, ambivalent, disorganized). Avoidance and ambivalence do not appear to be pathological forms of attachment. Disorganized attachment does appear to carry with it substantial developmental risk. We have found that the caregiving system framework helps to differentiate mothers of avoidant, ambivalent, and disorganized children according to whether their treatment of the child is organized in terms of caregiving or is overwhelmed by their own attachment needs and representations. Whether one views abdication of caregiving as pathological (i.e., linked to the child's developmental or mental health risk) or functional (i.e., permitting the mother to save herself) will depend on the level of explanation that one chooses.

As we review the points we have made in this paper, we see once again that, fundamentally, attachment theory and psychoanalysis are observing similar phenomena. By framing caregiving in behavioral systems terms, it is our hope that we can begin to move discourse about the mother toward a more common explanatory framework, one that is consistent with contemporary scientific views of behavior. Of course, this is precisely what Bowlby originally intended.

REFERENCES

Aber, L., Slade, A., Cohen, L. & Meyer, J. (1989), Parental representations of their toddlers: Their relationship to parental history and sensitivity and toddler security. Paper presented at the biennial meeting of the Society for Research in Child Development, Kansas City, MO..

Ainsworth, M. D. S. (1989), Attachments beyond infancy. *Amer. Psychol.*, 44:709–716.

———— Blehar, M. C., Waters, E. & Wall., S. (1978), *Patterns of Attachment: A Psychological Study of the Strange Situation.* Hillsdale, NJ: Lawrence Erlbaum.

———— & Eichberg, C. (1991), Effects on infant–mother attachment of mother's unresolved loss of an attachment figure, or other traumatic experience. In: *Attachment Across the Life Cycle*, ed. C. M. Parkes, J. Stevenson-Hinde & P. Marris. New York: Routledge, pp. 160–186.

Ammaniti, M. (1994), Maternal representations during pregnancy and early infant–mother interaction. In: *Psychoanalysis and Development: Representations and Narratives*, ed. M. Ammaniti & D. S. Stern. New York: New York University Press, pp. 79–96.

———— & Stern, D. (1992), *Attachment and Psychoanalysis.* Rome: Gius, Laterza, & Figli.

Anthony, E. J. & Benedek, T. (1970), Parenthood. In: *Psychology and Psychopathology*. Boston: Little, Brown.

Belsky, J. , Campbell. S., Cohn, J. & Moore, J.(1996), Instability of attachment security. *Dev. Psyc.*, *32*, 921–924.

Belsky, J. (1999), Patterns of attachment in a modern evolutionary perspective. In: *Handbook of Attachment Theory and Research,* ed. J. Cassidy & P. Shaver. New York: Guilford Press, pp. 141–161.

———— Rosenberger, K. & Crnic, K. (1995), The origins of attachment security: "Classical" and contextual determinants. In: *Attachment Theory: Social, Developmental, and Clinical Perspectives,* ed. S. Goldberg, R. Muir & J. Kerr. Hillsdale, NJ: The Analytic Press, pp. 153–184.

Benedek, T. (1959), Parenthood as a developmental phase: A contribution to the libido theory. *J. Amer. Psychoanal. Assn.,* 7:389–417.

Benoit, D. & Parker, K. (1994), Stability and transmission of attachment across three generations. *Child Dev.,* 65:1444–1456.

Bibring, G., Dwyer, T., Huntington, D. & Valenstein, A. (1961), A study of the psychological processes in pregnancy and of the earliest mother–child relationship. *The Psychoanalytic Study of the Child,* 16:9–24. New York: International Universities Press.

Blatt, S. J. & Blass, R. B. (1994), Relatedness and self-definition: A dialectic model of personality development. In: *Development and Vulnerability in Relationships,* ed. G. G. Noam & K. Fischer. Hillsdale, NJ: Lawrence Erlbaum, pp. 309–338.

Bowlby, J. (1969), *Attachment and Loss. Vol. 1: Attachment.* New York: Basic Books, 1982.

———— (1973), *Attachment and Loss. Volume 2: Separation.* New York: Basic Books.

———— (1980), *Attachment and Loss. Volume 3: Loss.* New York: Basic Books.

———— (1984), Caring for the young: Influences on development. In: *Parenthood: A Psychodynamic Perspective,* ed. R. S. Cohen, B. J. Cohler & S. H. Weissman. New York: Guilford Press, pp. 269–284.

Bretherton, I. (1985), Attachment theory: Retrospect and prospect. In: *Growing Points in Attachment Theory and Research,* ed. I. Bretherton & E. Waters. *Monographs of the Society for Research in Child Development,* 50:3–35.

———— Biringen, Z., Ridgeway, D., Maslin, D. & Sherman, M. (1989), Attachment: The parental perspective. *Infant Mental Hlth. J.,* 10:203–221.

Bus, A. G. & van IJzendoorn, M. H. (1992), Patterns of attachment in frequently and infrequently reading mother–child dyads. *J. Genetic Psychol.,* 153:395–403.

Carlson, E. A. (1998), A prospective longitudinal study of disorganized/disoriented attachment. *Child Devel.,* 69:1107–1128.

Cassidy, J. (1994), Emotion regulation: Influences of attachment relationships. In: *The Development of Emotion Regulation: Biological and Behavioral Considerations,* ed. N. A. Fox. *Monographs of the Society for Research in Child Development,* 59:228–249.

———— & Kobak, T. (1988), Avoidance and its relation to other defensive processes. In: *Clinical Implications of Attachment,* ed. J. Belsky & T. Nezworski. Hillsdale, NJ: Lawrence Erlbaum, pp. 300–326.

Cicchetti, D. & Carlson, V. (1989), *Handbook of Child Maltreatment: Clinical and Theoretical Perspectives.* New York: Cambridge University Press.

Cohen, R. S., Cohler, B. J. & Weissman, S. H. (1984), *Parenthood: A Psychodynamic Approach.* New York: Guilford Press.

Cole, M. & Cole, S. R. (1996), *The Development of Children.* New York: Freeman.

Cowan, C., Cowan, P., Heming, G. & Miller, N. (1991), Becoming a family: Marriage, parenting and child development. In: *Family Transitions, Vol. 2,* ed. P. Cowan & M. Hetherington. Hillsdale, NJ: Lawrence Erlbaum, pp. 79–108.

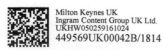

Milton Keynes UK
Ingram Content Group UK Ltd.
UKHW050259161024
449569UK00042B/1814